THE
PSYCHEDELIC
HANDBOOK

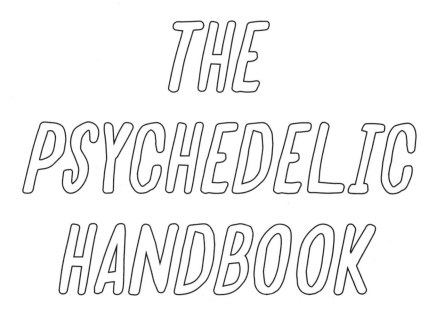

THE PSYCHEDELIC HANDBOOK

A Practical Guide to PSILOCYBIN, LSD, KETAMINE, MDMA, and DMT/AYAHUASCA

RICK STRASSMAN, MD

Published by:
Ulysses Press
PO Box 3440
Berkeley, CA 94703
www.ulyssespress.com

ISBN: 978-1-64604-381-1
Library of Congress Control Number: 2022932751

Printed in the United States by Kingery Printing Company
10 9 8 7 6 5 4 3 2 1

Acquisitions editor: Kierra Sondereker
Managing editor: Claire Chun
Editor: Scott Calamar
Proofreader: Renee Rutledge
Front cover design: Rebecca Lown
Layout: Winnie Liu

For Emily Ellingson, MD (1978–2010)

CONTENTS

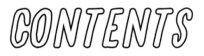

AUTHOR'S NOTE

This book is about the history and science of psychedelic drugs, as well as their uses, potential benefits, and risks in everyday life.

I ask the reader to consider all of the following cautions before using any of the information in my book.

PSYCHEDELICS USED IN THIS BOOK. My book is limited to discussions of psilocybin; LSD; mescaline, peyote, or San Pedro; ketamine; salvinorin A or *Salvia divinorum*; MDMA; 5-methoxy-DMT or the venom of the Colorado River/Sonoran Desert toad; ibogaine; and DMT or ayahuasca. At no point am I referring to prescription or illicit opiates; amphetamines or methamphetamines; nitrous oxide; alcohol; sedative-hypnotics; cannabis/marijuana; "bath salts"; cocaine; "research chemicals"; volatile inhalants such as gasoline, paint thinner, or glue; or any other drug not explicitly referenced here.

POSSIBLE POSITIVE HEALTH EFFECTS. Preliminary clinical research data suggest psychedelics have a role to play in treating a variety of mental health conditions, but none are yet approved by the US Food and Drug Administration except for a proprietary brand of ketamine in those with cases of treatment-resistant depression who are currently taking an antidepressant. While people who microdose find the practice helpful, there are no scientific data supporting these claims.

POSSIBLE NEGATIVE HEALTH EFFECTS. The use of psychedelics may result in negative psychological and/or medical health effects, and so does the discontinuation of medicines that you may be taking now if you wish to stop them before taking a psychedelic. Some of the potential side effects, risks, and drug interactions are discussed in detail in Chapters 3 and 11. As noted below, you should discuss the health risks of taking a psychedelic—and the best way to reduce those risks—with your healthcare provider. Not doing so can result in serious consequences, including emotional and mental problems such as anxiety, depression, suicidal thoughts, psychosis, and flashbacks.

CONSULT YOUR HEALTHCARE PROVIDER. Although I describe how psychedelics may interact with your health needs, including your medications, it is very important for you to consult your own primary care and/or psychiatric provider before using any psychedelics and before decreasing or stopping any medications that you may be using if you wish to do so before taking a psychedelic. The decision about whether to take a psychedelic is yours, but it depends on your own health issues. You should discuss the benefits and risks with a suitable healthcare provider before making a decision.

LEGAL RISKS. Possessing or consuming a psychedelic may lead to arrest and criminal prosecution. Most psychedelics are categorized under federal law as Schedule I controlled substances, the most restrictive class of drugs, and they are defined as "drugs with no currently accepted medical use, a lack of accepted safety for use even under medical supervision, and a high potential for abuse." Some states and municipalities have legalized and decriminalized these substances for personal use, but federal law supersedes state and municipal law, and state law supersedes municipal law. Therefore, that doesn't mean that possession of and/or using a psychedelic are entirely without legal consequences, including arrest and conviction for a crime. Before acquiring and/or using psychedelics, you must check with your local authorities—and consult an attorney—to determine what legal risks you are taking. The risk is even greater if you share these substances with others.

NO ENDORSEMENT. I have conducted extensive research for my book, and several of my sources are mentioned in the Acknowledgments and Recommended Reading. However, all of the opinions and advice in the book are mine alone, and no endorsement or affiliation with my sources is claimed or suggested.

GUIDING OTHERS. If you plan to use my book as a resource to help guide others, you should give all of these cautions to the people with whom you work.

PREFACE

The seeds for *The Psychedelic Handbook* first appeared in my childhood dreams. Dreams, much like psychedelic experiences, clarify for us feelings and thoughts that, while already existing in our minds, remain frustratingly obscure in the normal state of consciousness. Both psychedelics and dreams, therefore, are mind manifesting or mind disclosing—the traditional understanding of the word "psychedelic."

My dreams were of flying and its accompanying joy. There was a freedom and exhilaration, a newfound level of self-intimacy, and a riveting visual perspective of the world around me. So, when I had my first psychedelic experience in my late teens, it felt familiar. At the same time, I had to know more—both about the psychedelic experience personally and how psychedelics worked. From that point onward—through college, medical school, and psychiatric and clinical research training—I never lost sight of these long-term goals.

Substances that produce psychedelic effects are first and foremost chemicals—specific molecules with specific properties. Even in college, it was clear to me that chemistry was essential in understanding how psychedelics affect the mind. Chemistry always fascinated me, especially fireworks. Creating fireworks provided a satisfying intellectual challenge, the results of which were exciting displays of color, sound, and smell. There was the additional element of danger, treading on the edge of the forbidden in order to access fascinating sensations and thrilling emotions. I began college as a chemistry major, thinking I would become a fireworks magnate.

Family and friends dissuaded me instead to pursue medicine. However, I never completely gave up my love of brilliant colors and edgy feelings—I simply transferred their location from the outside world to the inside of the mind. This was how I made my way into psychedelic research. It is a classic case of "research is me-search."

Twenty years after my first psychedelic experience, one sunny and cold November day in Albuquerque in 1990, my dreams came true. This was when I administered the first dose of the powerful psychedelic drug DMT into the arm of a human volunteer in the General Clinical Research Center of the University of New Mexico. The US National Institutes of Health funded, and the FDA and DEA approved, this project—a series of rigorous psychopharmacology dose-response studies. We wished to determine what DMT and psilocybin did in a group of healthy human volunteers.

I had previously discovered the first known function of melatonin in humans in my search for a "spirit molecule." Now, with a pediatric neuroendocrinology professor helping guide this study's development, I applied the same psychopharmacological principles to examining psychedelic drug effects.

These studies began the renaissance in clinical research with psychedelics in the United States. Before I finished the project five years later, I had administered four hundred doses of DMT at various strengths to over fifty subjects. We also began administering psilocybin—the primary ingredient in magic mushrooms—to human volunteers. This was the first new American study with this compound as well. We gave psilocybin only twenty times, but in so doing generated preliminary data regarding effects of various doses and provided guidance for subsequent American studies with it. These protocols established the regulatory and scientific platforms that all subsequent American studies have used. In addition, the psychedelic drug effect rating scale we developed at UNM in the early 1990s continues in widespread use within the research world. Now, we see a veritable explosion of interest in psychedelic drugs: academic, scientific, media, religious, therapeutic, and commercial. An accessible, thorough, neutral, expert introduction to these compounds is thus timely.

Knowing about psychedelics and how best to use them requires more than simply scientific training. Also necessary is a multidimensional approach to the mind, and by extension, to the spirit. Aware of this, years before I began my New Mexico studies, I embarked upon several long-term involvements with spiritual and psychological disciplines.

Psychologically, I underwent a four-year course of classical psychoanalysis—the "gold standard" of Freudian psychotherapy—in my thirties. I laid on the couch, up to five days a week, with my analyst sitting (mostly) quietly behind me and to my side. This was the culmination of my interest and involvement in this type of self-examination that had begun a decade earlier as a medical student in the Bronx. During my analysis, I gained firsthand knowledge of the intense relationship that develops when one voluntarily enters a psychologically infantile, helpless, and dependent state for the sake of greater self-knowledge. I learned about the power of trust in a solid, tactful, empathic guide in helping navigate frightening and primitive memories and feelings. Later, I called upon this analytic role model when supporting DMT and psilocybin volunteers through their own, at times, confusing psychedelic experiences.

Spiritually, I was raised Jewish and had a bar mitzvah. However, I became involved in Buddhism in my early twenties, and studied and practiced for over twenty years under the supervision of one of the oldest Zen temples in the United States. I underwent lay ordination, and helped found and administer an affiliated meditation group for many years.

In my forties, I returned to my Jewish roots and began intensive Hebrew Bible study, which led to a book on psychedelics and Hebrew biblical prophecy.[1] This eighteen-year project required a deep dive into the Hebrew Bible,

---

1. Rick Strassman, *DMT and the Soul of Prophecy* (Rochester, Vermont: Park Street Press, 2014).

the Hebrew language, medieval metaphysics, and theology. Two excellent mentors graciously provided advice along the way: an academic Modern Orthodox rabbi and an Israeli professor of medieval Jewish philosophy.

My experience working with people extends beyond the world of research. During my eleven years in academics, I also treated psychiatric patients—inpatient and outpatient—in a variety of settings. After leaving the university, I worked solely in the clinical world for the next thirteen years in community mental health centers as well as in a private psychotherapy and psychopharmacology practice. This amounts to a quarter century of treating close to one thousand patients, ranging from the most regressed and psychotic murderers and drug addicts to high-functioning academics, white-collar professionals, and artists. My clinical skills served me well during my psychedelic research work, and my psychedelic research skills served me well in my clinical work.

Inside and outside the university, I have trained and mentored psychiatric residents in psychotherapy and psychopharmacology, medical students, and graduate students studying disciplines as varied as neuroscience and pastoral counseling. I have served as a peer reviewer and editor for manuscripts that scientists submit for publication in scientific journals and have authored or coauthored about fifty peer-reviewed scientific papers. In addition, I have consulted regularly to academic, government, commercial, and nonprofit entities for over thirty years.

My 2001 book—*DMT: The Spirit Molecule*[2]—has inspired a generation of psychedelic psychotherapists, researchers, and neuroscientists. *The Spirit Molecule* has appeared in over a dozen languages and sold a quarter million copies. It also was the inspiration for a successful documentary of the same name, which I coproduced, about the DMT research.

---

2. Rick Strassman, *DMT: The Spirit Molecule* (Rochester, Vermont: Park Street Press, 2001).

Finally, I know about these drugs. By various means and in various settings, I am personally familiar with the effects of every substance I discuss in this handbook.

My intention in describing my background—personal, academic, psychological, and religious—is to underscore my approach to the psychedelic drugs. I am not writing as an advocate or adversary of psychedelic drugs, nor am I a newcomer to the field. Rather, I do not believe that we know enough about what psychedelics do, how they do it, or their positive and negative potential to unequivocally come down on one side or the other. Therefore, my stance is to summarize what we do know, what we do not, and why it matters: scientifically, psychologically, and spiritually.

INTRODUCTION

In the 1950s and 1960s, psychedelics were the "wonder drugs" of psychiatry. They lifted psychiatry off the psychoanalytic couch and into the brain, ushering in the new discipline of psychopharmacology—how drug effects on brain chemistry change our consciousness. While antipsychotic and antidepressant medications also appeared at this time, psychedelics promised the greatest revolution in mental health care. Their allure included providing psychedelic-assisted psychotherapy for intractable emotional and addictive disorders, keys to unlock the secrets of psychosis, training aids to enhance empathy in psychotherapists, and a shortcut to creativity and spiritual enlightenment.

However, just as quickly as psychedelics' star rose, it fell. The social unrest of the 1960s—and the extent to which psychedelics contributed to this chaotic historical period—turned the public and government against them. Human use of psychedelics went underground, and the field of clinical research entered two decades of suspended animation. Now, once again, psychedelics are in the spotlight.

Everywhere we hear and read about a "psychedelic renaissance." Scientists at the world's best universities are avidly investigating psychedelics, and new academic centers dedicated to their study appear every few months, receiving tens of millions of dollars from enthusiastic philanthropists. This mainstreaming of psychedelics is drawing extraordinary venture capital, and dozens of new psychedelic startups are jockeying for position. Even at this early stage, several new companies have valuations of greater than $1 billion.

Swirling around these drugs are so many claims and counterclaims, hopes and fears, information and misinformation. How do we make sense of this groundswell of interest—scientific, cultural, media, spiritual, and commercial?

I begin this handbook with psychedelics' history. Many of these substances occur in the natural world, and Indigenous people have been using them for millennia; for example, psilocybin in "magic" mushrooms, DMT in ayahuasca, mescaline in peyote, 5-methoxy-DMT in toad venom, ibogaine in the iboga plant, and salvinorin A in *Salvia divinorum*. Modern Western psychedelic research began by identifying and isolating these compounds, and later characterizing and synthesizing them. Using these natural substances as building blocks, new synthetic psychedelics later appeared: LSD, ketamine, and MDMA.

Next, I provide a general description of how psychedelics make us feel— physically and emotionally, their effects on what we hear and see, our thought processes and sense of self. The altered states of consciousness psychedelics produce share features with other, nondrug, altered states like psychosis, dreams, and spiritual experiences. These similarities have led to the extraordinary number of names people have given these drugs. I will unpack these names and suggest that what we call psychedelics to a considerable extent determines what they do.

I discuss what we have learned about these drugs' potential benefits over the last fifty years, both therapeutic and as tools to enhance wellness. No drugs as powerful as psychedelics are only "good," however, and here I will also review adverse effects.

The next three chapters summarize what we know about how psychedelics work: biologically and psychologically. These "mechanisms of action" chapters provide me the opportunity to indulge in one of my favorite topics—medieval metaphysics—and how this ancient discipline may shed light on understanding the complex effects of psychedelics. And how about the "spiritual" properties of psychedelics? What are they, how do they come about, and how might our beliefs about them lead down a slippery slope of religious intolerance?

More than any other drugs, psychedelics bridge the mind-body gap. Their biological and psychological effects are impossible to separate. The biological effects of the drug modify our experience, and our experience modifies the biological effects of the drug. This leads us into the critical idea of "set and setting."

"Set" refers to who we are at the time of drug ingestion, and "setting" to where we take it. These two factors determine how any individual psychedelic drug experience takes its unique form. Experiences that are positive or negative, helpful or harmful, full of ideas or full of pleasure all turn on issues of set and setting. Set and setting may therefore help explain the panacea-like effects of psychedelics. Whatever we wish for them to do in either giving or taking them, they do.

I believe the set and setting phenomenon points to how psychedelics may help solve the mystery of the placebo response—how our beliefs and subjective experience modify our biology. One piece of this puzzle is exciting new research that demonstrates that psychedelics stimulate the growth of new neurons in the brain as well as increasing the complexity of their connections. These are psychedelics' "psychoplastogenic" effects.

Next, I write about individual psychedelic drugs—their history, botany, pharmacology, usual doses, and how one takes them. I will review each drug's time course, unique psychological and/or biological effects—including adverse ones—and their legal status.

Any handbook must, by definition, provide practical how-to advice. This book's longest chapter therefore does just that. While neither I nor Ulysses Press advocates taking drugs nor breaking the law, there are those who are curious enough to venture into this territory to accept the attendant risks. Therefore, it is important to do everything possible to maximize benefit and minimize negative outcomes. In that chapter I will also address the growing public awareness of sexual and other types of abuse at the hands of those who administer psychedelics in various settings.

Microdosing—taking non-psychedelic doses of a psychedelic—is increasingly popular. I will summarize what we know, and more to the point, what we do not know, about microdosing. The legal landscape of psychedelics is rapidly changing, and the next to last chapter will help you navigate current trends in "decriminalization" and "legalization." In my concluding remarks, I underline my intention for writing this handbook— that is, as an educational resource—and share my enthusiasm for future developments in the field.

PART I

WHAT ARE PSYCHEDELIC DRUGS?

CHAPTER 1

WHAT ARE PSYCHEDELICS?

Psychedelic drugs are remarkable mind-altering substances, arguably the most interesting drugs in all of medicine. Some compare their effects to schizophrenia and other psychotic disorders, others to near-death and spiritual experiences, even alien abduction. They reliably produce a unique state of mind in which you see visions and hear voices. You may lose awareness of your body while your consciousness travels through deep outer—or inner—space. You may feel almost unbearable ecstasy, terror, or both—or nothing at all. New ideas, feelings, and insights flood your mind. You may encounter and interact with intelligent beings who inhabit the "psychedelic space"; these "beings" may heal, instruct, and love; or they may be hostile and threatening. No matter what their specific effects might be, the hallmark of any full psychedelic experience is the sense that it is "more real than real." Effects of some psychedelics begin seconds after smoking or injecting them, and some last up to eighteen hours after consuming them orally.

HISTORY

Psychedelic mushrooms, plants, and even animals play a vital role in the religious and social lives of Indigenous societies, especially those in the

Americas. We are only now beginning to recognize the depth and practical applications of this wisdom. Part of our relative ignorance regarding Indigenous use is suppression by the Catholic Church after the Spanish conquest of Latin America in the 1500s. Concerns about "witchcraft" and "paganism" overrode any scientific, medical, or anthropological curiosity. Remnants of this intolerance remain to this day.[3]

Modern psychedelic drug research began with the isolation of mescaline from the peyote cactus by German chemist Arthur Heffter in the 1890s. This plant is the most important religious sacrament of the present-day Native American Church in North America,[4] but its use dates back to at least the time of the Aztecs. Mescaline research, however, did not make much headway in the world of psychiatry at the time. Its gastrointestinal side effects were unpleasant, but perhaps more important was Freud's hold on psychiatry in the first half of the twentieth century. The founder of psychoanalysis, despite his well-documented use of cocaine as a mental stimulant, had little interest in religious and spiritual issues. He saw them as representing psychopathology, and successful treatment did away with "infantile" tendencies or experiences rather than working to bring them about. While a few papers reported mescaline's ability to enhance psychotherapy, its association with "primitive" psychological states and cultures prevented wider acceptance.

Freudian psychology began falling out of favor after World War II. It was slow, expensive, and questionably effective—features that led psychiatry to seek new models and treatments for mental illness, especially for veterans returning from the war. The discovery of LSD's effects in the mid-1940s, therefore, came at an especially fortunate time.

_____

3. A prominent American psychiatrist once referred to this stance as "pharmacological Calvinism." This alludes to the belief that we must prescribe and take drugs only to treat illness, rather than to also use them for pleasure, creativity, or spiritual purposes.

4. More about this in Chapter 7.

Albert Hofmann, a chemist working at Sandoz Pharmaceuticals (now Novartis) in Basel, Switzerland, synthesized LSD in the late 1930s. However, he learned of its mind-altering effects only several years later when he accidentally ingested it. LSD fired the imagination of both the public and science because of its amazing potency—active at doses of millionths of a gram—and its effect on serotonin in the brain. In fact, these latter effects led to the identification of serotonin as the first neurotransmitter.[5] LSD thus opened the door to the new science of psychopharmacology—how drugs affect the mind.

For the next several decades, LSD and related compounds revolutionized our understanding of how the brain works. They also demonstrated great promise in benefiting a host of difficult-to-treat conditions: depression, addiction, autism, sociopathy, pain, and end-of-life despair.

These promising lines of research were of little help, however, after LSD escaped the laboratory. Its widespread use amplified the social unrest of the 1960s, especially against US military involvement in Vietnam. In addition, while research use of psychedelics was quite safe, uncontrolled use was wreaking havoc within the general population. Reports of adverse effects—suicide, violence, birth defects, chromosome damage, and psychosis—began accumulating. Poorly prepared and marginally psychologically healthy youth were taking unknown quantities of unknown drugs in combination with alcohol and other substances in unpredictable settings. Emergency rooms and psychiatric wards were filling up with "LSD casualties." A public health emergency was underway. It could not help that former Harvard psychologist and LSD researcher-turned-advocate Timothy Leary urged tens of thousands of protesters at this time to "turn on,[6] tune in, and drop out," as well as overthrow the prevailing political structure.

---

5. Neurotransmitters are chemicals that allow adjacent nerve cells to communicate with each other. More on neurotransmitters in Chapter 4.

6. That is, take psychedelics.

Within academics, contention also existed. Some research groups touted these drugs as "spiritual," "transpersonal," and capable of producing "mystical experiences." This segment of the psychedelic research world continues influential, as we see by the belief that "mystical experiences" explain psychedelics' beneficial effects. In addition, the psychiatric and nonpsychiatric use of the term "entheogen"—"generating God within"—reflects this continuing and controversial mingling of science and religion. It was getting difficult to tell the difference between psychiatric research and the development of a religious cult. This mixing of science and religion did not reassure federal regulators and the National Institutes of Health—who funded much of the early American psychedelic research.

NEFARIOUS USE

The 1950s and 1960s also saw the intelligence and military establishments of the US and other countries use psychedelics as potential chemical warfare agents. In these settings, there were few ethical constraints and minimal or no informed consent. The American government set up prostitution houses and dosed subjects unknowingly to determine if LSD and other compounds might function as a "truth serum." Another approach was to disperse psychedelic drugs as nonfatal debilitating agents, and yet another was to employ them as brainwashing tools.

None of these approaches was successful. LSD effects were too unpredictable to serve as useful "truth serums" in unwitting subjects. Testing in American service members demonstrated mixed results as debilitating agents, but the greater problems were geographic and climactic variables that made dispersion difficult. Attempts to create more effective killers using LSD as a brainwashing tool failed because of the importance of subjects' preexisting personality. That is, it was not possible to turn a peace-loving person into an assassin. On the other hand, if one already harbored assassin-like goals and values, LSD might not even be necessary.

THE CONTROLLED SUBSTANCES ACT OF 1970

This perfect storm of controversy, politics, public health, and black ops gone wrong resulted in Congress passing the Controlled Substances Act (CSA) of 1970. This law, by virtue of its multiple firewalls, effectively extinguished human studies with these drugs. Nevertheless, their underground use continued at about the same levels after the CSA as before it. Adverse effects have greatly diminished, however, because people in the twenty-first century usually take lower doses. They also can call upon fifty years of accumulated wisdom regarding how to take psychedelics more safely, as well as how to care for those having difficulties.

While clinical research ground to a halt, basic science in lower animals continued, as the regulations for nonhuman research were significantly less burdensome. As a result, our increasing understanding of the pharmacology of LSD and other psychedelics—especially their relationship to the serotonin neurotransmitter system—has been responsible for the development of more effective and less toxic psychiatric and neurological drugs for a variety of conditions: depression, psychosis, headache, and nausea/vomiting.

SET AND SETTING

The most important lesson that we learned during the first wave of psychedelic enthusiasm was the crucial role of "set" and "setting" in determining the results of any particular drug experience. This concept helps explain why the same drug at the same dose given to different people in the same circumstances produces different responses. It also helps explain why the same drug at the same dose given to the same person in different circumstances produces different effects. This is a topic I emphasize regularly throughout this handbook. So, let us introduce it here.

"Set" refers to the state of the person who takes the psychedelic. This includes their physical and mental health. Is someone ill, on multiple medications, drinking excess alcohol, or abusing opiates? Or is that person healthy—do they exercise daily, make certain to get adequate sleep, and maintain a healthy diet? How about current depression, panic attacks, or even simply dealing with multiple life stressors? Or are they happy and fulfilled—possessing a supportive social network and enjoying their work? Have they taken psychedelics before, and if so, what was their experience? Ecstatic travel through the cosmos or a horrifying descent into the netherworld?

Set also includes expectations and intention. What do they expect will happen, what are their goals, what are their hopes and fears? Do they wish for their cancer to disappear or to accept the reality of a rapidly approaching death? It also includes one's beliefs about psychedelics themselves, what they call them, and how that reflects beliefs about what psychedelics do and how they do it. Are they "entheogens"—generating the divine within? Are they "psychotomimetics"—producing a time-limited psychosis? Or are they "psychedelics"—manifesting or disclosing what already exists in a person's mind, simply awaiting greater clarification?

"Setting" refers to the environment in which one takes the psychedelic. Indoors or outdoors. With friends or alone. In a research or party environment. It also includes the set of everyone with whom one experiences the drug effect. Thus, a host of interpersonal factors come into play. Are they friends, antagonists, or neutral parties? Scientists, therapists, or spiritual brethren? Why are they taking and/or giving someone psychedelics and what do they expect will happen? What do they want in return?

HUMAN RESEARCH RESUMES

Clinical studies with psychedelics slipped into two decades of hibernation after the CSA and similar international laws took effect. The tide began shifting in both Europe and the US in the late 1980s. A German paper appeared in 1989 documenting a clinical mescaline study, and my work with DMT at the University of New Mexico began shortly thereafter. The New Mexico research created the necessary regulatory and scientific procedures for other American groups to begin their own work with these drugs. These included psilocybin for obsessive-compulsive disorder at the University of Arizona, MDMA in normal volunteers at UCLA and Wayne State, ibogaine at the University of Miami, and psilocybin at Johns Hopkins University. The latter project, because of its emphasis on spiritual experience, has been especially effective in capturing public attention.

A new generation of more open-minded federal regulators and funders is reviewing requests for psychedelic research more favorably than has been the case for decades. Many of these individuals have had their own positive psychedelic experiences and want to see more research take place. In addition, fifty years allows the chaotic and inglorious downfall of psychedelics to fade from memory. We also continue facing psychiatry's limited success in treating a multitude of emotional ills, many of which are the same conditions for which psychedelics appeared to be uniquely promising in the 1950s and 1960s. The mental health toll of the ongoing COVID pandemic has magnified the pressing need for better and more widely available options for care. Psychedelics may offer hope that other treatments do not.

TYPES OF PSYCHEDELIC DRUGS

While I go into detail regarding each psychedelic drug in later chapters, here I wish to introduce important general terms.

"Classical psychedelics" belong to one of two major groups of chemical compounds: the tryptamines and the phenethylamines.

DMT, 5-methoxy-DMT,[7] and psilocybin are tryptamines. They all possess in their chemical structure a molecule of tryptamine. Tryptamine is an amino acid that plants make by themselves, and which animals produce by chemically modifying dietary tryptophan. Beginning with this tryptamine core, nature attaches other components, such as methyl groups; for example, adding two methyl groups to tryptamine results in "dimethyltryptamine," or DMT. The human body synthesizes DMT and perhaps also 5-methoxy-DMT. Botanical DMT is the visionary ingredient in the increasingly popular Amazonian brew ayahuasca. 5-methoxy-DMT is the active ingredient in "toad venom," which the Sonoran Desert toad produces, and which people smoke for its effects. Psilocybin, from a large number of "magic mushrooms," exists only in fungi.

In the world of psychedelic chemistry, as everywhere else, there are lumpers and splitters. Here, I will take the side of the lumpers, and call both LSD and ibogaine tryptamines. The splitters will say that LSD is an ergoline, a more complex chemical category. You can see tryptamine in the LSD molecule, however, and therefore placement in the general tryptamine family is common. LSD is synthetic, a product of chemically modifying ergot, a mold that grows on several grains. The African psychedelic ibogaine, like LSD, incorporates a tryptamine molecule into its larger, more complex structure, and likewise we can call it a tryptamine.

The other family of classical psychedelics is the phenethylamines, of which mescaline from the peyote cactus is the most famous. Amphetamine and

---

7. Or "5-MeO-DMT."

methamphetamine, which are not psychedelic, are also phenethylamines. MDMA belongs to this category; however, it is not a classical compound like mescaline.

The synthetic compound ketamine belongs to a completely different family—the arylcyclohexylamines—as does the closely related drug of abuse PCP.

Salvinorin A from *Salvia divinorum*—"diviner's mint"—also belongs to a distinct molecular category. In fact, it is unique among the psychedelics because it is not a nitrogen-containing alkaloid. Instead, it is a terpene, a large family of molecules that is essential to the field of natural products like fragrances and colorings. Turpentine, for example, is a terpene.

PHYSICAL EFFECTS[8]

Classical psychedelics increase heart rate and blood pressure, but when people take them by the oral route, the effects are not especially dramatic. However, when the route of administration is injection, smoking, or snorting, as in the case of short-acting tryptamines like DMT, these cardiovascular effects can be profound and potentially dangerous in someone with heart disease.

The increase in body temperature that occurs with classical drugs is not dangerous, but that which MDMA causes can be. This is the reason MDMA

---

8. The following two sections—"Physical Effects" and "Psychological Effects"—refer primarily to the classical psychedelic drugs. Other compounds in this handbook—MDMA, ketamine, and salvinorin A—share many but not all features of the classical compounds. I will highlight those differences when discussing each "nonclassical" compound in subsequent chapters. Nevertheless, there are more similarities than differences among the various substances. In addition, while we are learning more about the psychedelic effects of marijuana/cannabis, it does not appear in this handbook. However, to the extent that cannabis may produce psychedelic effects, much of what I say here is also relevant to it.

is sometimes fatal when people take large quantities in hot, crowded dance venues without drinking fluids that also contain vital electrolytes.

Pupil diameter uniformly increases with classical compounds, and this may contribute to light sensitivity and blurred vision. Nausea and/or vomiting may occur with any psychedelic but are usually short-lived except with ayahuasca and mescaline-containing peyote. Goose bumps are not unusual and may accompany the onset of effects—the "hair-standing-on-end" anticipation that marks initial stages of the psychedelic experience.

PSYCHOLOGICAL EFFECTS

Psychedelic drugs affect every aspect of human consciousness: perception, body awareness, emotions, thinking, and sense of self. In this way, they differ from compounds that modify only one or two mental functions.

When lecturing, Alexander "Sasha" Shulgin, the father of modern psychedelic chemistry, referred to three types of psychoactive drugs. The ↑ ("up") compounds are the stimulants like amphetamines, caffeine, and cocaine. These increase energy, mood, and concentration. The ↓ ("down") drugs are the sedative-hypnotics: alcohol, benzodiazepine antianxiety agents like Xanax and Klonopin. They sedate us and slow our movements and thoughts. Then there are the ★ ("star") substances—the psychedelics— that affect every aspect of consciousness.

Sensory elements often predominate during the psychedelic drug experience. What we look at is brighter or duller, may shift in shape or melt, become larger or smaller. With eyes open—and especially closed— we observe colorful, geometric, swirling, kaleidoscopic images, or more or less recognizable inanimate and animate objects. What we hear may be gentler or harsher, louder or softer. We hear sounds emerging from the silence—voices, mechanical noises, singing, the wind, or echoes.

Psychedelics often cause synesthesia—the blending of two sensory modalities. The most frequent example is "seeing sounds." Music may produce colors we see in our minds or even in the "external" world. Less frequent is a blending of other sensory modalities; for example, "hearing" things that normally we just see with our eyes.

Our body feels different—hot or cold, light or heavy, bigger or smaller. Our skin is more or less sensitive, and our senses of taste and smell change in pleasurable or displeasing ways. We may lose complete awareness of our body, and our consciousness appears to inhabit a disembodied state.

Emotions dry up or overflow, wax and wane, are overpowering or absent. We experience two opposite feelings at the same time: happiness and sadness, anxiety and tranquility, terror and ecstasy. We might resolve long-standing emotional difficulties. We feel what others feel, or altogether lose our empathy.

Our thinking becomes clearer or more confused, faster or slower. New ideas and insights may pour forth, we might get stuck in repetitive thinking, or we may stop thinking entirely. Time passes more slowly or rapidly—five minutes may feel like years, and hours seem to pass as swiftly as just a few minutes.

Psychedelics modify our sense of self and that self's ability to interact with the inner and outer worlds. We may feel more or less in control of ourselves, or experience others influencing us in positive or negative ways. The ability to determine our own lives has never felt more convincingly clear, or we see the inevitability of uncaring fate. We have never felt our individuality so strongly, we may forget who we are, or we merge with a white light outside of time and space.

Once acute drug effects end, and if it has been a "successful experience," there is often a "psychedelic afterglow." This is a feeling of ease, contentment, confidence, energy, clear thinking, and elevated mood. It may last for days and occasionally for weeks.

Perhaps the most striking overall effect of psychedelics is what one of my mentors, Daniel X. Freedman, called "portentousness." Ido Hartogsohn has recently coined the term "meaning-enhancement." Both refer to an all-consuming, overarching conviction that what one is experiencing is "more real than real." This does not mean that the visions and the voices take on a greater reality than things we see and hear in normal everyday consciousness. Rather, the meaning of the experience, its significance, intensity, personal relevance, and truth value are greater than anything we have normally felt or believed.

THE NEAR-DEATH AND ALIEN CONTACT EXPERIENCES

There are similarities between the near-death experience (NDE) and psychedelic drug effects, especially those of ketamine and DMT. These include disembodied consciousness, the conviction that one has died, travel through a tunnel with a light at the end, and a world full of beings. When comparing descriptions of the NDE with psychedelic drug states, one study found DMT to be the most similar, whereas another pointed to ketamine. The similarity between the DMT state and the NDE has led researchers to study the biology of the dying brain. Recent data suggest that DMT levels rise after cardiac arrest in rodents, especially in the visual cortex. Therefore, we have supporting data suggesting a role for endogenous DMT, which the body itself naturally produces, in generating some of the features of the near-death experience.

When I began my DMT research, I had little interest or knowledge regarding the alien contact experience. However, the frequency of "encounters with beings" in my volunteers forced me to consider the overlap in descriptions of these two sets of experiences. For example, in both there is an inner pressure and vibration just before breaking through to contact with beings, one's physical body drops away upon entering the "alien" space, and the beings themselves are powerful and intelligent. In both, a variety of intense interactions with beings take place, interactions that are convincingly real. There are, of course, no physical signs of "contact," and this led me to suggest that there may be a type of alien contact experience in which the interactions are only "consciousness to consciousness" rather than "body to body."

Psychedelic drugs modify every component of consciousness. This is why, unlike other psychoactive substances, psychedelics possess such a bewildering collection of names. These names, what they mean, and what they say about our beliefs regarding psychedelic drug effects, are the subject of our next chapter.

CHAPTER 2

THE MANY NAMES FOR PSYCHEDELICS: WHY THEY MATTER

My interest in studying psychedelic drugs began by noticing similarities between descriptions of the psychedelic drug state and those resulting from certain types of meditation. This suggested to me that meditation might release a naturally occurring psychedelic substance in the brain, or that both psychedelics and meditation activate the same brain areas. In either case, similar subjective experiences would result. Likewise, other nondrug-altered states share features with the psychedelic drug effect: psychosis, prophecy, alien abduction, and the near-death experience. And everyone dreams—a nightly entry into a world possessing many psychedelic features. To the extent that the psychedelic state and any of these other syndromes overlap, one could propose a common biological denominator.

The similarities between psychedelic drug effects and other naturally occurring altered states has led to an abundance of names for these substances. Before I vote for "psychedelic" as the best term, I will review how other names came about and discuss their limitations. In this way, I hope to make my point about the superiority of the term "psychedelic."

HALLUCINOGEN, PSYCHOTOMIMETIC, AND SCHIZOTOXIN—PSYCHEDELICS AND PSYCHOSIS

"Hallucinogen" was the most popular medical-legal term for decades. However, not all psychedelic experiences involve visions and voices, and not everyone agrees as to the exact meaning of "hallucination." In addition, we rarely consider the things we see on psychedelics as objective as everyday reality, which is a characteristic of a "true hallucination."[9] At the same time, psychedelic experiences are deeply meaningful, and to refer to them as hallucinations slights that significance. It implies our experience is unreal, imaginary, somehow pathological or deranged.

"Psychotomimetic" is a closely related term. It reflects the belief that psychedelics cause a "model psychosis"—a time-limited psychotic state similar to schizophrenia. Symptoms common to both syndromes include "disordered thinking," "paranoid delusions," "disturbed body image," "loss of self-identity," "abnormal emotional reactions," and so on. This notion was so dominant in early psychiatric research that rating scales for LSD in the 1950s and 1960s emphasized these types of effects to the exclusion of nearly all others. To the extent that any particular drug produced "psychotic experiences," researchers deemed that drug "LSD-like."

The psychotomimetic concept produced another name for psychedelics: "schizotoxic" or "schizotoxin"—alluding to the belief that they were psychosis-generating toxins, much like our use of "neurotoxin" today to describe certain drugs' detrimental effects on the brain.

---

9. The exception is salvinorin A, which may cause people to interact with hallucinated objects and run the risk of injuring themselves or others.

How valid is the model psychosis idea? It depends. It depends on the type of psychosis and the particular symptoms of the disorder. For example, with respect to the hallucinations and delusions of schizophrenia, especially the acute paranoid type, classical psychedelics' effects share features. With respect to "burned out" schizophrenics, those who frequently inhabited the back wards of state mental hospitals, they are not a good model. On the other hand, ketamine seems more likely to mimic certain aspects of the withdrawn catatonic state that occurs with this group of patients.

Keep in mind, too, that the circumstances of the psychedelic drug state and schizophrenic syndromes vary considerably. Someone who takes LSD might have similar symptoms to someone with acute schizophrenia. However, they willingly took a drug, know that their symptoms are the result of drug ingestion, and that the effects will resolve in several hours. Someone suffering the same symptoms for weeks, months, or years, however, must adapt to their presence. These adaptations then become an essential part of the person's psychology—their behavior and beliefs. Temporary suspiciousness solidifies into complex enduring paranoid delusions. In addition, schizophrenics may have underlying neurological and cognitive deficits that can limit the adaptations possible in response to long-term "psychedelic" symptoms.

A number of theoretical and practical applications grew out of the model psychosis concept. For example, if researchers could identify the biological effects of the "psychotomimetic" LSD—say, abnormalities in neurotransmitter function—this might point to the existence of similar malfunctions in nondrug psychotic conditions. Those neurotransmitter abnormalities might then be modifiable with medication, in much the same way that SSRI antidepressants correct abnormal serotonin function in depression.

This was a particularly busy research area after the discovery of naturally occurring DMT in human body fluids. Scientists sought abnormalities in the DMT system in psychosis: overproduction, ineffective breakdown, or hypersensitivity to the effects of normal amounts. Before human studies ceased in 1970, scientists were even developing antibodies against DMT as a potential antipsychotic treatment.

While new American research with classical psychedelics has not focused on the psychotomimetic model, European groups continue to employ this framework.

These theories also provided a rationale for administering psychedelics to psychotic patients in the 1950s and 1960s. How similar were the visions and voices caused by DMT or LSD to those that take place in "everyday" psychotic experience? To the extent that they resembled each other, this would support the idea that a naturally occurring psychedelic was responsible for the symptoms of schizophrenia. Perhaps, then, anti-psychedelic drugs might be useful antipsychotics.

The evidence supporting a relationship between psychedelics and endogenous psychosis during the first wave of studies was inconclusive. By the time scientists had refined their understanding of the similarities and differences between the two syndromes, clinical research was over. With the renewal of human studies, researchers are again administering psychedelics to schizophrenics; however, only ketamine has seen use this way, not classical compounds. It appears that ketamine increases psychotic symptoms in schizophrenic patients that are no different from their "everyday" symptoms. Similarly, then, anti-ketamine drugs may prove effective in clinical practice.

The psychosis-psychedelics connection raised two additional avenues of research during the first wave of human research.

One involved psychotherapy with psychotic patients. These were usually long-term back ward residents of state mental hospitals. Psychiatrists hoped that these oftentimes mute, immobile, intensely preoccupied patients might increase their engagement with the outside world after taking a psychedelic. The results were mixed—some did and some did not.

The other research area was training therapists who worked with psychotic patients. Here, the belief was that inducing a "time-limited psychosis" in clinicians would increase their empathy. They would know "firsthand" what it was like to be psychotic—hearing and seeing things that others normally do not, experiencing a fragmented sense of self, and relating to the world in a paranoid and disorganized manner. While this strategy makes sense, there were few if any publications addressing its actual effectiveness. I believe it deserves a reexamination.

ONEIROGEN: PSYCHEDELICS AND DREAMS

Oneirogen comes from the Greek *óneiros*- "dream" and *gen*- "to create." An oneirogen produces a state similar to dreaming. This term is relatively rare both within the scientific and lay psychedelic communities. I have seen it mostly in the context of ibogaine, but whether ibogaine's subjective effects are distinct from those of the other classical compounds is uncertain.

There are many areas of overlap between the psychedelic and dream states: "visions"; "voices"; existing in a nonphysical world; highly altered senses of self, space, and time; memories of long-forgotten events; and symbolic representation of usually unconscious conflicts or wishes.

When considering accounts of big psychedelic experiences, it is difficult to avoid making an association with dreams. During our DMT studies, when listening to one of our volunteers describe his drug session, the attending nurse said, "That sounds just like my dreams." And, when reviewing my book *DMT: The Spirit Molecule*, one writer suggested that the title be changed to *DMT: The Dream Molecule*.

While descriptions of the two states overlap considerably, I believe there are at least two ways to distinguish them. The most obvious is that a psychedelic experience takes place while awake, and dreams occur during sleep. Another difference is more subtle and relates to the reality sense each possesses. Responding to the nurse's comment comparing her dreams and his DMT experience, our volunteer said, "That was a dream you described; this is real. It's totally unexpected, quite constant, and objective. One could interpret your looking at my pupils [which we did to measure their diameter] as being observed, and the tubes in my body [for blood sampling and drug administration] as the tubes I'm seeing in my visions. But that is a metaphor, and this is not at all a metaphor. It's an independent, constant reality."

Nevertheless, the overlap between the psychedelic and dream experiences is undeniable. And, with the discovery of high levels of DMT in the mammalian brain, one of the most interesting questions now is whether levels rise during the dream state.

ENTACTOGEN AND EMPATHOGEN

These are relatively new terms for MDMA-like drugs. Entactogen is a combination of the Greek root *en-* meaning "within" and the Latin root *tactus-* meaning "touch," and refers to these drugs' ability to put people in closer contact with themselves, especially their emotional lives. Empathogen—"generating empathy"—emphasizes their empathy-enhancing effects. The two terms are interchangeable because they describe the same family of compounds and their predominant emotional effects.

ENTHEOGEN AND MYSTICOMIMETIC: PSYCHEDELICS AND SPIRITUAL EXPERIENCE

"Entheogen" is a relatively new and increasingly popular term for these drugs. It neatly expresses three concepts in one word. *En-* meaning "within," *theos-* "God," and *gen-* "to produce." Thus, entheogens "generate God from within." These ideas, therefore, require us to consider the nature of spiritual experience itself, a term that possesses considerable ambiguity. To the extent that we can agree on a common vocabulary, we are that much further ahead in tackling these thorny issues.

Let us begin with the term "spiritual." This refers to thoughts, feelings, or images that possess the highest qualities of the mind. Similar terms are "holy," "sacred," "religious," and "pure." "Spiritual" differs from the "everyday," "profane," "bestial," or "carnal." "Spiritual" may also refer to things that are immaterial, incorporeal, or invisible. It may refer to the immaterial nature of humans—their soul or spirit. More specifically, "spiritual" may concern God, God's spirit or word, or the soul upon which God acts.

A "religion," on the other hand, is a system of beliefs that expresses the relationship between the spiritual nature of humans and the spiritual world. This involves a sense of responsibility, dependence, awe, reverence, fear, and love. It also includes specific concepts, feelings, imagery, music, and practices that flow from these beliefs. A religion may contain or channel spiritual thoughts, feelings, imagery, and impulses. However, spirituality frequently exists outside of traditional religious institutions. This is what people mean when saying they are "spiritual but not religious."

I like to divide spiritual experiences into two types: the "mystical-unitive" and the "interactive-relational." In both, we are dealing with an altered state of consciousness with spiritual characteristics. Either or both may occur within or outside a religious tradition. Within a religious tradition, we may call them "religious experiences," and they partake of imagery, vocabulary, and concepts consistent with that religion.

The hallmark of a unitive-mystical experience is "unity," what some refer to as "ego-dissolution." There is no longer an individual sense of self, no inner or outer, no object or subject, and one's consciousness merges with "God," "the ground of all being," "pure awareness," the "white light," a formless content-free powerful "reality." Buddhists call this phenomenon "emptiness," out of which all existence emerges, but which itself is empty of anything specific or identifiable. Time and space no longer exist. There is a certainty and truth—the conviction that what one is experiencing is "more real than real"—a positive mood, and "ineffability." This last term refers to the sense that one cannot describe the state verbally.

In contrast, an interactive-relational spiritual experience is full of content, there is the maintenance and even strengthening of one's sense of self, time and space continue—although in a somewhat modified way—mood effects are more variable, and the state is full of information, often verbal. Like the mystical-unitive state, there is also the feeling that what one is witnessing is more real than real.

William James was a Harvard psychologist at the turn of the nineteenth century who wrote the famous *The Varieties of Religious Experience*. His notion of the mystical-unitive as the highest form of spiritual experience came about as a result of his relationship with the Indian religious figure Swami Vivekananda. The two became acquainted when Vivekananda presented the idea of a "universal religion" at the Parliament of the World's Religions in Chicago in the late 1800s. The notion that a fundamental religious experience underlay all of the world's major religions appealed to James, and he incorporated this idea into his famous book. By doing so, he wished to emphasize the similarities among religious traditions, hoping this might lead to less sectarianism and strife.

However, this universal religion of Vivekananda was a specific one; that is, Vedanta Hinduism. And, the notion of an underlying religious experience common to all traditions is not true. One need only look at the Hebrew Bible (Old Testament) tradition of prophetic experience. There are no examples of a mystical-unitive state in this entire collection of twenty-four books. Rather, the prophetic experience is solely interactive and relational. Take a look at Chapter 1 of Ezekiel, where the heavens open and the prophet witnesses a host of celestial beings, spinning wheels, rotating spheres, fire, and ice. Stunned, he falls to the ground, and an angel lifts him, thus beginning a verbal dialogue between human and the divine.

Nevertheless, there is a widespread notion of a universal spiritual experience—"hardwired" into the human species—that psychedelics activate. This idea dominates discussions of the spiritual effects of psychedelics within and outside academics.

This has had two unfortunate effects. One is that it establishes a goal for any particular psychedelic session. That is, if someone taking a psychedelic—and those administering it—values the attainment of a mystical-unitive state, a sense of disappointment results on both sides if they fail to do so. A more pernicious result is the belief that interactive-relational spiritual experiences are inferior to mystical-unitive ones. This is an opinion, a theological stance, and lacks supporting evidence.

Comparing unfavorably the interactive-relational experience with the mystical-unitive one results in regarding unfavorably religious traditions for whom the interactive-relational experience is fundamental; that is, the basis of their tradition. As Judaism is the most well-known religion basing itself on the interactive-relational—that is, prophetic—experience, this has resulted in Jewish beliefs sitting in the crosshairs of psychedelicists—academic and lay—who promote the universal mystical-unitive state.

I've digressed into different types of spiritual experience because of the increasing popularity of calling psychedelics "entheogens," a practice that emphasizes the notion that psychedelics are inherently spiritual. This is like asserting that psychedelics are somehow inherently "schizotoxic." Neither is true. Rather, psychedelic effects result from who gives them, who takes them, and why; that is, set and setting. And this is why "psychedelic" is the best term, as I will suggest shortly.

There are practical limitations to "entheogen," too. Not everyone who takes psychedelics seeks a spiritual experience, and emphasizing these effects may cause those who might otherwise benefit from a psychedelic session to shy away. In addition, the presence of "theos" points to the existence of God, divinity, and a spiritual world, which many people do not believe in. It also assumes that God—if one believes in God—exists within us, rather than outside of us. This, too, is a belief that not everyone shares, including those who may wish to use a psychedelic drug for spiritual reasons. Finally, the idea that a drug can generate God suggests a metaphysical model that traditionally religious individuals might object to.

PSYCHEDELIC: MIND MANIFESTING OR MIND DISCLOSING

I prefer the term "psychedelic." It is the most generic and therefore the most inclusive. This is a crucial point, because one may take a psychedelic for any number of reasons in any number of settings. The drugs themselves don't "produce" psychosis any more than they "produce" spiritual experience. Rather, they simply interact with the mind of the person taking them.

"Psychedelic" is a Greek word consisting of two roots. *Psyche-* refers to the mind, soul, or intelligence. *Delos-* means to manifest, reveal, disclose, or make clear or understandable. This word captures the essential features of the psychedelic state. Previously invisible or hidden contents of the mind are now visible.

Stanislav Grof, the father of modern LSD psychotherapy, proposed that psychedelics are nonspecific amplifiers of unconscious mental material. We can expand this notion by saying that they also impact conscious contents. That is, if one is already more or less aware of particular thoughts and feelings, they may become clearer, more true, meaningful, and significant. Better and more beautiful.

Anglo-Canadian psychiatrist Humphry Osmond originally coined the term, but it fell out of favor because of its association with countercultural movements of the 1960s. In addition, popular media co-opted the term—trivializing it—to refer simply to an aesthetic: a type of music, fashion, or art. Over time, however, the cultural baggage that "psychedelic" carried for so long has become much lighter. The term now appears more often than any other in lay and scientific settings

AGAIN, SET AND SETTING

What one chooses to call psychedelics turns on what properties they wish to emphasize, and what—in the research setting—rating scale the research team uses. And their name feeds back onto what their effects are, and especially how we interpret them.

Consider this situation: Someone volunteers for a study with a "psychotomimetic" drug. Staff treat the intoxicated volunteer as if they were schizophrenic, and after the drug effect has worn off, the volunteer fills out a "schizophrenia rating scale." Now, consider this situation: That same person volunteers for a study with the exact same psychedelic drug, but in this case, researchers call it an "entheogen." Staff treat the intoxicated volunteer with reverence, respect, and compassion, and then administer a "spiritual experience rating scale." It's not difficult to see how different such experiences will be with the same drug in the same individual in such strikingly different settings.

Each of these approaches—the psychotomimetic or the entheogenic—possesses merits. However, we must not confuse two important concepts: the effects of the drugs themselves and the purposes for which one is using them. One might use psychedelics to study psychosis just as one might use them to induce a spiritual experience. However, there is a crucial difference between the essential properties of the drug and the wished-for or expected outcome.

This is why I believe "psychedelic" remains the best term. It avoids overlaying interpretive schemes onto their essential feature—which is to manifest and disclose the mind's contents.

CHAPTER 3

WHAT ARE PSYCHEDELICS GOOD FOR? WHAT ARE THEIR RISKS?

In this chapter, it may seem as if I emphasize negative effects of psychedelics more than positive ones. It is not my intention to paint psychedelics in a negative light but to provide a balanced perspective regarding potential risks and potential benefits. It is not difficult to find glowing accounts of the results of psychedelic drug use, both within and outside the research environment. These are real reports dealing with real data. On the other hand, with the rush of enthusiasm regarding psychedelics, I advise caution in too quickly dismissing psychedelics' potential adverse effects. These rarely receive anywhere near the attention that more promising ones do.

POTENTIAL BENEFITS

In the 1950s and 1960s, research demonstrated a host of positive findings regarding classical psychedelics' effects. Most projects utilized LSD, while a few studied psilocybin, mescaline, or the DMT-like compounds DET (diethyltryptamine) and DPT (dipropyltryptamine).

Then, as now, psychiatry was disappointingly ineffective in treating common yet disabling conditions: alcohol and opioid addiction, depression, anxiety, pain, end-of-life despair, autism, and antisocial and other personality disorders. Most studies, although not as well designed scientifically as they are today, indicated benefit from psychedelic drug administration. In addition to treating mental illness, some research demonstrated enhancement of creativity in scientists and artists. Spiritually oriented studies with psychedelics during the first wave of enthusiasm were rare. The most well known was the Marsh Chapel Good Friday Experiment at Boston University, in which theology students on psilocybin had more profound religious experiences than those who took placebo during a Good Friday service.

Current psychedelic-assisted psychotherapy studies address all the just-mentioned conditions and include ones about which we had not yet established diagnostic clarity and/or awareness of their prevalence. These include tobacco dependence, post-traumatic stress disorder, obsessive-compulsive disorder, and eating disorders like anorexia nervosa and bulimia nervosa. We also now have ayahuasca in our psychedelic toolbox. Research suggests that acute administration of this DMT-containing brew is effective for the same disorders for which other classical compounds are. In a longer-term setting, people use ayahuasca tea regularly over many decades in churches where it serves as a sacrament, and evidence suggests benefit across a large number of mental and physical health categories.

Studies with newer nonclassical compounds like MDMA and ketamine have produced similarly promising results in treatment-resistant depression, alcoholism, post-traumatic stress disorder, and social anxiety.

One of the most remarkable aspects of current research is the demonstration that benefits for anxiety, suicidality, and depressive symptoms begin quickly, within an hour or two after drug administration. With ibogaine, drug craving and withdrawal symptoms likewise respond very quickly. Interestingly, this rapid time course corresponds to the induction of neurogenesis (new nerve growth) and neuroplasticity (more nerve cell connections) in lower animals and in test-tube studies.

While psilocybin has been the classical psychedelic drug most researchers are now using, I believe this is due to political considerations and not any unique properties of the drug.[10] The pharmacology of LSD and psilocybin is similar, as are their subjective effects. Neither is the argument persuasive that psilocybin's shorter duration of action than LSD's provides a distinct advantage. Practically speaking, what is the difference between a six-to-eight-hour drug session and an eight-to-ten-hour one? Both require a full day at the clinic or hospital. Rather, psilocybin's current popularity is mostly due to its lesser notoriety than LSD as a drug of abuse. In addition, the widespread availability of psilocybin mushrooms, as well as their being "natural entheogens" increases the drug's appeal to researchers who advocate for wider access to psychedelics in general. Decriminalization and legalization proponents have been quick to exploit these researchers' implicit advocacy.

Psychedelic-assisted psychotherapy in the 1950s and 1960s took two approaches. One model was the psycholytic, in which patients took low but psychedelic doses of the drug in the setting of long-term treatment, usually Freudian psychoanalytic psychotherapy or psychoanalysis. This was a regular part of one's treatment; that is, patients might receive psycholytic doses of LSD, say, once a month in the setting of years-long therapy. These patients were not especially ill, usually suffering from neurosis or a personality disorder. The scientific rigor of this work was significantly less than studies that used higher doses of psychedelics in academic settings, and results rarely appeared in scientific journals.

The other model was the psychedelic, where therapists administered a small number of high doses of drug. Here, the goal was to attain a "peak,"

---

10. This is also one of the reasons I chose the relatively obscure DMT and not LSD for my initial research projects.

"psychedelic," or what we now call "mystical," experience. This is today's predominant approach. There is, however, a growing consensus supporting the value of combining traditional psychotherapeutic modalities with high-dose psychedelic drug sessions, thus utilizing the best of both models. These therapies include motivational interviewing, cognitive behavioral therapy, psychoanalytic psychotherapy, and client-centered approaches.

Of note were a handful of studies giving psychedelics daily for the treatment of mood disorders, in a model like what one sees in daily antidepressant treatment. The acute psychedelic effects faded rapidly because of tolerance while the antidepressant responses were substantial.

Recent enthusiasm for classical psychedelic-induced spiritual experiences—that is, using psychedelics for nonmedical purposes—has also led to studies demonstrating that psychedelics increase "wellness." For example, they help meditation; contribute to a more open, accepting, and compassionate personality; and increase clergy's dedication to their profession.

"Field studies" involve administering questionnaires to people taking psychedelics in non-research settings; for example, toad venom smoking circles and ayahuasca retreats. In addition, researchers use internet surveys to look for relationships between psychedelic drug use and other variables. These studies suggest that psychedelics improve creativity and alter metaphysical beliefs; and that psychedelic users have better cardiovascular health and less diabetes than nonusers, are less lonely, are less likely to use cocaine, are more likely to remain out of jail after release, are more progressive politically,[11] have a greater appreciation of nature, and have better domestic relationships. However, one such study, while suggesting an association between psilocybin use and less depression, also found more depression in those who used LSD.

---

11. However, neo-Nazi groups also use psychedelics to cement their own sets of beliefs and justify their actions.

One must view these survey studies with caution, however, because they do not establish a causal relationship. In other words, we do not know that psychedelics cause these effects. It may be that those who are already in better cardiovascular health take psychedelics more often than those in poor cardiovascular health, or those who already appreciate nature take psychedelics more often than those who do not.

POTENTIAL RISKS

The following discussion addresses the classical psychedelics. I will address adverse effects of nonclassical drugs in subsequent chapters.

PHYSICAL RISKS

Classical psychedelics are physically nontoxic. I am unaware of any deaths that these pure compounds or uncontaminated plants have caused when people do not mix them with other substances. Reports of birth defects and chromosome damage contributed to the anti-psychedelic backlash of the late 1960s, but better-designed follow-up studies disproved those early claims. In addition, there is no convincing evidence that classical psychedelics produce brain damage, reduce IQ, or cause other neurological adverse effects. While a study in the 1970s suggested lower scores in LSD users on a test of memory, a more recent article indicated ayahuasca users scored higher on that same test.

ADDICTION

"Addiction" is a complex notion and involves the interrelated phenomena of tolerance, withdrawal, dependence, and craving. It also straddles physical and psychological categories of adverse effects, which is why I place it here—between physical and psychological risks.

"Tolerance" refers to closely spaced repeated use of a drug producing fewer effects over time. Consequently, a higher dose is necessary to produce the same results. In the case of classical psychedelics, tolerance occurs rapidly. For example, taking the same dose of LSD every day for three or four days abolishes psychological effects of the original dose. After about the same number of abstinent days, sensitivity returns to normal. "Cross-tolerance" refers to tolerance to different drugs of the same class. Someone tolerant to LSD will not respond to psilocybin as robustly as someone who is not tolerant to LSD, nor will someone tolerant to psilocybin respond normally to mescaline.

"Withdrawal" refers to physical and psychological symptoms accompanying abrupt cessation of drug use. Caffeine withdrawal is mild whereas alcohol withdrawal may be fatal. The withdrawal syndrome produces symptoms opposite of the acute drug effect. For example, when someone withdraws from the sedating drug alcohol, they are hyperexcitable and may develop seizures. Stopping psychedelics does not produce a physical withdrawal syndrome, even after daily dosing.

"Dependence" may be psychological or physical. For example, one may be dependent on a benzodiazepine sleeping pill to get a good night's sleep. However, they take the drug as prescribed, do not combine it with other drugs like alcohol, and do not keep raising the dose. However, abrupt cessation will produce a physical withdrawal syndrome. And once withdrawal is over, some may find that they were psychologically dependent on the drug—they "crave" it. This means they spend inordinate time thinking about and wishing they could obtain and use the drug. However, even without physical dependence causing physical withdrawal symptoms upon cessation of use, some may depend upon a drug psychologically, which likewise leads to craving and drug-seeking.

"Addiction" is a medical-psychiatric disorder in which one cannot stop using a drug despite negative consequences—health, vocational, or social. One can be tolerant to a drug (fewer effects with the same dose) and undergo withdrawal when stopping (physical dependence) but may not be addicted to it. For example, someone is taking an opiate that a physician is prescribing for an acute injury, requires higher doses for the same pain relief after a week or so, and once stopping the drug, experiences opiate physical withdrawal. However, they do not crave the drug, nor continue taking it beyond the prescribed time.

If someone continues using psychedelics despite the drugs causing problems, one may consider them addicted. They wish to return to the same state repeatedly to cope, or to reinforce beliefs that no one else shares. This is a psychological, not physical, addiction and is quite rare. Keep in mind, too, that daily dosing of classical psychedelics abolishes their effects, so compulsive daily use does not occur. An exception is that tolerance to DMT—and probably 5-methoxy-DMT—does not develop with repeated administration, so out of control use, while infrequent, does occur.

PSYCHOLOGICAL RISKS

In the adverse effect literature from the 1950s through the 1970s—the period from which we have the most information—there were two sets of data. One was from normal volunteers and psychiatric patients who received psychedelics in academic or private psychotherapy settings. The other consisted of articles describing patients who presented to emergency rooms or psychiatric hospital units suffering ill effects of these drugs.

In carefully screened, supervised, and followed-up research and/or therapy subjects, the risks resulting from psychedelic drug administration were extraordinarily low. The rate of psychosis lasting more than twenty-four hours was approximately 0.1 percent, and suicide attempts 0.1 percent or less; i.e., five attempts in 25,000 sessions. Both rates are comparable to or lower than what one sees in the general population.

On the other hand, the "LSD casualties" about which the media and politicians raised the alarm—psychotic breaks, suicides, and violent behavior—occurred in individuals taking unknown amounts of unknown drugs in unsupervised settings, in combination with alcohol or other substances. Oftentimes they also carried a predisposition to negative reactions—having a personal or family history of mental illness.

Adverse Effects or Challenging Experiences?

As a physician, I am familiar with and readily use the terms "adverse effect" or "adverse reaction." A penicillin-induced rash is an adverse reaction to the drug. Likewise, a fatal disturbance of one's heart rhythm resulting from a bronchodilator is an adverse reaction. These are generic terms that encompass a wide spectrum of phenomena. Adverse effects are unintended negative consequences of drug exposure.

However, just as terms like "entheogen" glorify potential benefits of psychedelic drugs, renaming adverse effects "challenging experiences" minimizes their risks. Both are examples of creating new terms for these drugs and their effects—positive and negative. Their purpose is to promote certain beliefs about psychedelics rather than provide information about what they are and what they do. While this approach to the positive and negative effects of psychedelics is part and parcel of the psychedelic subculture, it has gained legitimacy through psychedelic researchers' publications; for example, developing and promoting a "challenging experience questionnaire" to characterize adverse drug effects.

Is short-lived anxiety at the onset of a psychedelic session a challenging experience? How about a rash from penicillin? Medically and psychiatrically, these are mild, short-lived adverse effects. Is a chronic unremitting psychosis requiring long-term hospitalization and powerful antipsychotic medication a challenging experience? Likewise, a fatal arrhythmia from a bronchodilator is hardly "challenging." Medically and psychiatrically, they are severe adverse reactions with catastrophic outcomes.

"Challenging experiences" may provide comfort to those who are dealing with brief mild adverse effects and minimize undue concern about their consequences. However, the term does a disservice by providing false comfort to those suffering more dramatic adverse reactions by making it less likely that they seek necessary care. "After all, it's just a challenging experience."

"Short-," "medium-," or "long-term;" "mild," "moderate," or "severe"—these are all terms we use in describing negative effects of any drug in psychiatry and medicine. I see little reason to abandon them in the service of "psychedelic newspeak." On the contrary, the term "challenging experiences" may contribute to a backlash against psychedelics. Astute journalists could argue that researchers have become advocates instead of neutral scientists by using such expressions to minimize the existence of serious adverse psychological reactions.

For classical and nonclassical compounds, we can propose a continuum of adverse reactions. These may include brief anxiety, suspiciousness, or confusion in the context of the acute drug experience. These symptoms may continue and/or develop after drug effects have worn off. The most common are intense anxiety/panic reactions that resolve on their own within a day. Longer-lasting—one or two days—disturbances such as depression, anxiety, paranoia, or confusion also usually clear up by themselves or with modest support. Anything persisting for longer than a day or two should be cause for concern.

Psychedelics and Mental Illness

In most cases, psychedelics trigger mental illness in someone with a predisposition, either from a previous episode of, say, bipolar disorder, panic attacks, or schizophrenia, and/or because of a family history of such conditions. The psychedelic drug acts like any other traumatic event that may trigger an acute episode of a serious psychological disorder. Other examples of potentially traumatic triggers of mental illness include marriage or divorce, going away to college or the military, or the death of a family member. Once such illnesses occur, regular treatment for the diagnosed disorder, regardless of what brought it on, is usually adequate. For example, one would treat a psychedelic-triggered manic episode in the same way as if psychedelics played no role. At the same time, it is important for that person to stop using psychedelics to prevent another occurrence.

Particularly troubling are situations in which people have taken enormous quantities of psychedelic drugs for prolonged periods. They may suffer from extraordinarily stubborn hallucinations and, especially, delusions. They frequently lack insight into the abnormal nature of their beliefs and experiences and are thus resistant to treatment. As a result, they will not refrain from further psychedelic drug use, which only prolongs and/or worsens their condition. We were aware of these cases in the early years of widespread psychedelic use, and they continue to surface nowadays.

Over the last twenty years I have received about a half dozen emails from concerned friends or relatives asking for help for someone they know who has overdone their psychedelic drug use and is now either in jail or a psychiatric hospital. This syndrome may be occurring at a lower rate now because of the accumulated wisdom of the last fifty years in averting serious adverse effects—using lower doses and getting help more quickly when troubles arise. However, with psychedelics' increasing popularity and easier accessibility resulting from decriminalization and legalization movements, we may be in for more of these tragic cases.

Flashbacks, Post-Hallucinogen Perceptual Disorder, and Reactivations

The original term "flashback" appeared in the 1960s to describe the reoccurrence of certain aspects of the psychedelic drug experience after resolution of acute effects. It is convenient to divide them into "perceptual," "physical," and "emotional" categories that may alternate and/or overlap with each other. The modern psychiatric term for these experiences is "post-hallucinogen perceptual disorder," but this is not especially useful because perceptual effects are only one aspect of a broader syndrome. An even more modern term is "reactivation." While not as troubling a renaming of psychedelic drug effects as "entheogenic" and "challenging," I do not believe it adds anything to the discussion. And to the extent that "flashback" draws attention to post-traumatic stress disorder—a condition that may be useful in explaining how these symptoms occur and how to treat them—"flashback" remains the most suitable name.

Flashbacks are not rare. Data from early research indicated that they occurred in up to 77 percent of those who had at least one psychedelic drug experience. They may be more frequent in those who have taken more psychedelics, at higher doses, for a longer period, but this is not a consistent finding. Flashbacks also may occur more frequently after especially traumatic experiences with these drugs.

Flashbacks are usually mild and time-limited, especially if one avoids psychedelics and other mind-altering drugs after they emerge. Some people enjoy the "free trip" that flashbacks represent. However, they may be particularly troublesome in a small minority of people, interfering with normal activities. In these cases, there are no reliable effective treatments, and even long-term abstinence may have negligible effect.

The causes of flashbacks are unclear. They do not result from lingering drug in the body. Neither does there seem to be an association between any personal and/or family history of psychiatric disorders making one predisposed to their development. There is no convincing evidence for brain damage. One theory borrows from the PTSD literature. Feelings— for example, fear—that were prominent during the psychedelic/traumatic state will trigger other elements of that experience. Likewise, finding oneself in a situation—for example, a traffic jam—in which the psychedelic/traumatic experience took place will bring about a recurrence of other aspects of what happened during the original event.

ADVERSE EFFECTS OF THE SETTING

While I have discussed the adverse effects of the drugs themselves, it also is important to consider potential adverse effects of the setting in which one takes psychedelics. We can divide these into two categories. One is unscrupulous practitioners—those who administer psychedelics more for their own benefit than the benefit of those they give them to. Another is the model within which one takes a psychedelic. These are not cut-and-dried distinctions, however, and the two may overlap. This topic is so important that I return to it in Chapter 11: How to Trip.

Unscrupulous Practitioners

Whether in group or individual settings, some who administer psychedelic drugs do not have the best interest of their charges in mind. They may manipulate, abuse, or otherwise take advantage of someone in a psychedelically induced vulnerable and suggestible state. For any healing, therapy, growth, or other significant changes to occur during a supervised drug session, trust is the essential bedrock of the relationship between those who administer and those who take a psychedelic.

There are several ways in which unscrupulous practitioners may take advantage of those who have placed their trust in them: sexually, physically, emotionally, spiritually, or financially. Even in a group setting with no clearly defined leader or guide, I have witnessed episodes of abusive behavior—psychological sadism, and racial, religious, gender, and ethnic slurs. The aftereffects of any such experiences can be profoundly unsettling and difficult to bring out in the open, like how difficult it is to report and deal with the consequences of rape. One factor making it so hard to sound the alarm is the charisma of the perpetrators, their standing in the psychedelic community—spiritual, academic, or therapeutic—and the gaslighting and blame projecting that they often invoke as their first line of defense. "It's nothing, you're overreacting." "You're imagining it." "It must be some problem you have." "They seduced me." "I was only doing it for their benefit." And so on. We are now witnessing a welcome frankness of discussions of this phenomenon.

Adverse Effects of the Model

Before we knew about the crucial role of set and setting in determining psychedelic drug effects, some research teams approached their use as sole pharmacological "chemotherapeutic" agents, like an antibiotic. For example, a normal volunteer, or even someone in a psychotherapy project, might find themselves in a padded seclusion room, tied down to a gurney, with bright overhead lights beaming down on them. A white-outfitted nurse peeked through a little window into the room at the hapless LSD-intoxicated individual, yelled a few questions through the door, scribbled notes on the clipboard, and disappeared for another two hours. As you might imagine, those studies did not go well.

Now, we are seeing almost the opposite situation taking place regarding adverse effects of setting. That is, the research team's expectations and beliefs about psychedelics—in this case, their "entheogenic" rather than their "chemotherapeutic" effects—collide with the "psychedelic" ones. By this I mean the conflict that arises when someone's experience under the influence of a psychedelic does not fit into the model's assumptions and the corresponding beliefs of the model's adherents. There are fine lines between guidance, direction, constraining, and coercion.

In a recent study of psilocybin-assisted psychotherapy for the terminally ill at Johns Hopkins University, a patient committed suicide after receiving a tiny non-psychoactive dose of psilocybin in the "placebo" part of the project. Both the university and FDA concluded that this was not an "adverse effect of psilocybin." However, I believe this is an example of an adverse effect of the model.

The Baltimore group utilizes the mystical experience model, believing that attaining a specific questionnaire-quantified psychological goal is how psychedelics heal. Preparation of subjects emphasizes the benefits of the mystical state, providing advice on how to attain it during the drug session, and therapists guide acute drug effects in such a way as to optimize its occurrence. The music selection steers the experience toward this goal as well, and integration occurs through the lens of the mystical experience belief system.

Imagine, then, the disappointment and demoralization in a dying patient who received a non-psychoactive dose of drug hoping for spiritual and psychological healing by a mystical experience. This is what most likely led him to commit suicide eleven days after his session. Perhaps if there were less (or no) emphasis on having a mystical experience, the outcome would have been different. Instead, he and his therapists would simply have worked with whatever material came up, rather than deal with the mutual disappointment that no such highly sought-after "breakthrough" occurred. A multidisciplinary "psychological autopsy" would be highly informative and could help prevent future similar tragedies.

Another potential adverse effect of a model is when someone trips in a highly alien context. This may happen when traveling to Latin American ayahuasca retreat centers that base their work on Indigenous shamanic models—beliefs and practices—that have little to do with where one comes from and to where one is returning. While this model might make sense at the time, deep in the jungle, integration of the experiences upon reentering one's normal, urbanized North American or Western European setting can be extraordinarily difficult.

In addition, an unscrupulous practitioner in a confusing setting might take advantage of a doubly disoriented individual on a psychedelic. The most common cases we hear about in this regard are when a shaman in the jungle sexually abuses someone in the course of their participation in an ayahuasca retreat. Reasons given may vary, but include things like: "In my culture, shamans like me become greater healers when we have sex with our clients." Or, "The spirit of ayahuasca told me that for your healing, you must give me $25,000 for my retreat center."

As I mentioned in the beginning of this chapter, I have found myself emphasizing potential adverse effects of psychedelics more than their potential benefits. There is no shortage of information regarding how helpful psychedelics are, but less obvious is where to turn to learn about their potential risks. Whenever one decides to take a psychedelic trip—for pleasure, spiritual purposes, brain imaging, or psychotherapy—informed consent is essential. You must know as much as you can about what you are signing up for. I hope that this exploration of the less glamorous side of psychedelics helps balance your appreciation of what is involved in a truly informed decision.

PART II

HOW DO PSYCHEDELICS WORK?

CHAPTER 4

HOW PSYCHEDELICS WORK: THE BRAIN

When considering how psychedelic drugs produce their effects, I like to use the term "mind-brain complex." On one hand, we experience drug effects in our minds: visions, voices, extreme emotions, and out-of-body travel. These are subjective experiences. On the other hand, psychedelics are drugs. They generate a host of biological responses—especially, but not only, in the brain. In some mysterious way, a process of translation occurs between these biological effects and subjective experience. The relationship between the brain and our mind is undeniable but inexplicable.

Drugs affect the brain and our conscious experience, and our experience affects the brain. What we think and feel activates some brain functions and inhibits others. This is especially the case with psychedelics. For example, if we react with fear when we lose awareness of our bodies, that fear modifies brain function differently than if we respond to that same bodily dissociation with joy. The profound effects of psychedelics on both our brain and mind, and the nature of their interdependency, provide powerful tools in studying consciousness itself.

Our current understanding of the mind-brain complex points to the importance of open-mindedness in discussing how psychedelics work. We know what they do biologically and psychologically, but we do not understand how biological changes translate into their extraordinary subjective effects.

This uncertainty plagues the entire field of consciousness research, an uncertainty that scientists call the "explanatory gap." This gap exists between physical processes in the brain—chemical, electrical, and magnetic—and subjective experience. Philosophers and neuroscientists alike cannot say for sure that we will ever bridge that gap.

We know, for example, that LSD attaches to receptors on specific nerve cells in the brain, and this in turn begins a series of downstream effects on other nerves, nerve centers, and connections among those centers. However, we do not know how—or why—these effects result in the subjective experience of a "trip."

HOW PSYCHEDELICS GET INTO THE BRAIN

Psychoactive substances must first make their way into the brain before exerting any effect. Nearly always, this is via blood that enters the brain. The exceptions are injection of a drug into the cerebrospinal fluid—a cushioning, nutrient-rich fluid that bathes the brain and spinal cord—via a spinal tap,[12] or directly into the brain itself. I do not recommend either!

How, then, to begin this process of getting a drug into the bloodstream? That is, what are the various "routes of administration"?

These include the oral route (swallowing), sublingual (under the tongue), buccal (packing into the cheek), rectal (as a suppository or enema), transdermal (applying directly onto the skin), subcutaneous (injecting

---

12. This is a medical procedure where one inserts a needle between two vertebrae in the lower back, puncturing the spinal canal. After gaining access to the cerebrospinal fluid, one may take a few drops for chemical analysis and/or inject drugs directly into the spinal canal.

under the skin), insufflating (snorting through the nostrils), smoking (vaporizing and then inhaling), intramuscular (injecting into a muscle), and intravenous (injecting into a vein). Several drugs are active by more than one route. For example, people may take ketamine orally or sublingually; or by snorting, smoking, rectally, or injecting. Most compounds, however, have one preferred method of administration; for example, the oral route for LSD and the smoked method for 5-methoxy-DMT.

Oral administration is the slowest way for drugs to enter the system, and it provides the smoothest onset and offset, as well as the longest duration. This is the preferred route for most of the compounds in this handbook. Onset is usually fifteen to sixty minutes, and absorption is often better with an empty stomach. Most orally active psychedelics exert their effects over two to twelve hours, and sometimes, as with ibogaine, even longer.

Sublingual, rectal, and buccal routes are faster than the oral one. Effects begin within a few minutes. This is a useful method for taking substances that stomach acid or liver enzymes would otherwise break down before entering the bloodstream, rendering them ineffective. Rectal use also eliminates the nausea and vomiting that can occur with noxious-tasting substances like mescaline-containing San Pedro cactus tea. Absorption of ketamine lozenges is buccal and sublingual and sees use in treating depression or pain in a medical setting.

The buccal route is rare as a primary method of administration. It occurs with salvinorin A when using fresh *Salvia divinorum* leaves rolled up in a quid and packed into a cheek. While the swallowed *Salvia* juice is not effective, absorption across mucous membranes of the cheek is.

Subcutaneous and intramuscular injection are quicker yet—onset within a couple of minutes. However, there is variability in the effectiveness of these methods, depending on blood flow and fat content of the injected tissue. It also requires proper injection technique, pure drug, and sterile equipment. Recreationally, it is easier to snort or smoke a drug than to inject it. However, some ketamine users like the intramuscular method (IM) because its one-hour duration is appealing. The IM route for ketamine is also common in medical settings for depression treatment.

Snorting is also quite rapid, and effects usually begin within a few minutes. Recreational users of ketamine snort the drug for a rapid and brief high. In addition, a proprietary ketamine spray—Spravato—is increasingly popular for outpatient treatment of depression. While most people smoke tryptamines like DMT and 5-methoxy-DMT, some snort water-soluble salts of these compounds.

Vaporizing a drug and inhaling its vapor—what we usually call "smoking"— and intravenous administration are the most rapid ways of getting a drug into your bloodstream. Smoking is the preferred route of administration for the short-acting tryptamines and salvinorin A. Effects begin within a few heartbeats. Smoking carries its own drawbacks. Coughing and poor smoking technique may limit how much drug one gets into the lungs. Breakdown of the drug by heat may occur, and the lung effects of smoking drug vapor may be detrimental. The rapidity of onset of smoked drugs can also produce disorientation that cuts short inhaling an effective dose.

The surest and most efficient route of administration is intravenous injection. This is how we administered DMT in the New Mexico research. Effects begin within a couple of heartbeats and peak between two and five minutes. Those with experience smoking DMT described the intravenous route as a half step more rapid. In addition to the technical requirements of intravenous injection, the purest and cleanest form of the drug is also necessary.

Once a drug makes its way into the blood, it still must get into the brain. The brain is highly selective about what it lets into its confines, strictly regulating entry through the "blood-brain barrier." This consists of tight-fitting cells that line blood vessels serving the brain. This functions to keep out water-soluble drugs—a property of the lipid, or fat layer, that surrounds these blood vessels.

For a drug—or any other substance—to cross the blood-brain barrier, there are two primary mechanisms. Lipid-soluble substances like alcohol and general anesthetics enter through diffusion, where they make their way from an area of higher concentration to one of lower concentration. The other mechanism—for water-soluble compounds—is active transport, where the brain expends energy to draw in that substance across the blood-brain barrier. Active transport occurs when the brain requires that substance, such as glucose for fuel. Interestingly, DMT is a compound that the brain actively transports into its confines, suggesting that the brain needs it for normal function.

PSYCHEDELICS AND NEUROSCIENCE

Once a psychedelic drug enters the brain, how does it cause the unique mental changes so many people seek? The visions, voices, ecstasy, and insights require changes in the mind-brain complex's function.

I approach the biological, pharmacological, and brain-imaging studies that scientists use to understand psychedelics' effects with two important considerations in mind. One of these is the reaction of readers to the "hard science" in my DMT book from 2001, when we knew relatively little about psychedelics' effects on human brain function. Even with the limited amount of information then available, readers got bogged down in my discussion of neurotransmitters, receptors, and psychopharmacology. They either skipped over this material—which was my advice—or stopped reading the book altogether. With that as a warning, if the following information appears meaningless and/or too technical, please skip over it and move on to the next chapters.

Another consideration is a realistic assessment of the power of "brain science" to tell us why psychedelic drug effects are so compelling, and how to use them for the greater good. In other words, so what if psilocybin reduces the activity of the brain's "default mode network"? Or, that there is a relationship between psychedelic-induced "ego dissolution" and certain changes in brain function? As we will see, these objective data simply confirm what careful subjective analyses already reveal about psychedelics' effects. The more important issue, at least for me, is how we use the psychedelic drug experience for our and others' benefit. At the same time, I do not want to disrespect the groundbreaking research now taking place. Rather, I wish to keep the "gee-whiz" factor in perspective.

That being said, there are practical consequences of ongoing high-tech studies. They will help us develop new psychedelics that target specific brain areas that mediate particular mental functions. For example, if we wish to develop a more visual or emotional psychedelic, drugs that turn on visual or emotional parts of the brain are candidates for such compounds.

In addition, to the extent that subjective effects of psychedelics overlap with those occurring in nondrug altered states—such as dreams or schizophrenia—we will gain insight into how these altered states come about. In the case of psychiatric illnesses, these data may lead to new treatments. That is, when brain function changes resulting from psychedelics overlap with those we see in psychosis, drugs that reverse those psychedelic-induced changes may prove useful in treating psychosis. Finally, we may learn how to modify brain activity without drugs using, for example, electrical, ultrasonic, or magnetic energy to induce "psychedelic" effects in the brain.

PHARMACOLOGY

Pharmacology is the study of drug effects on biological systems. With drugs that affect the brain, this becomes neuropharmacology. When dealing with how drugs affecting the brain influence behavior and subjective experience, we now have neuropsychopharmacology; in the case of humans, psychopharmacology is the more common term.

Let me introduce some fundamental concepts.

Neurons are nerve cells, and the ones that concern us are in the brain. Other nerve cells exist in the spinal cord and throughout the body—the gut, skin, muscles, and endocrine glands. There are approximately one hundred billion neurons in the human brain—the same number of stars as in the Milky Way. Neurons communicate with each other using neurotransmitters. These are chemicals that cross the synapse, a minuscule space between nerve cells. A typical synapse is between 20–40 nanometers across, much smaller than anything we can see with the unaided eye. By way of comparison, the width of a human hair is about 100,000 nanometers. There are approximately 2–3 trillion synapses in the human brain; that is, 2,000–3,000 billion synapses.

When two neurons communicate, we specify a presynaptic neuron and a postsynaptic one. The presynaptic neuron releases the neurotransmitter into the synapse. The neurotransmitter crosses the synapse and attaches to the postsynaptic neuron. We know of several dozen neurotransmitters, but for our purposes, there are a handful that concern us: norepinephrine (or noradrenaline), dopamine, serotonin, GABA (gamma amino butyric acid), glutamate, and endorphins—opiate-like substances that the brain makes.

After the presynaptic neuron releases its neurotransmitter into the synapse, that neurotransmitter binds to receptors on the postsynaptic neuron, like a key fitting into a lock. There are multiple subtypes of receptors for each neurotransmitter; for example, the serotonin (5-HT) type 2 and the dopamine (DA) type 1. Many of these subtypes possess their own subtypes; for example, 5-HT2A. Every neurotransmitter produced in the brain has specific receptors to which it binds.

A neurotransmitter either stimulates the postsynaptic neuron, inhibits it, or otherwise modifies its function—for example, its response to other neurotransmitters. A stimulated postsynaptic neuron now becomes a presynaptic one and releases its own neurotransmitters onto nearby neurons. Imagine, then, the vast web of neurotransmitter activity coursing through the brain at any given moment.

Once a neurotransmitter does its work, there are three ways that its effects end. One is by the presynaptic neuron reabsorbing that neurotransmitter, vacuuming it back up—what we call reuptake. Thus, the SSRI antidepressants like Prozac are "selective serotonin reuptake inhibitors." They interfere with reuptake of serotonin from the synapse back into the presynaptic neuron that originally released it. By reducing serotonin reuptake, SSRIs allow for more of the neurotransmitter to remain in the synapse and prolong its effects on the postsynaptic neuron.

Another way of clearing the synapse of neurotransmitters is metabolism—breaking them down into inactive byproducts using enzymes. This is how the body breaks down any substance—beneficial or harmful; for example, drugs by liver enzymes, protein by gut enzymes, or air pollutants by lung enzymes. One enzyme, monoamine oxidase type A (MAO-A), breaks down DMT extremely rapidly in the gut when swallowed, which is why oral DMT is inactive. In combination with a MAO inhibitor, as in ayahuasca, oral DMT remains in the gut long enough to make its way into the bloodstream and from there to the brain. Finally, neurotransmitters may simply be flushed out of the synapse, a process we call diffusion.

Neurotransmitters regulate elements of consciousness. We usually learn what those functions are by observing effects of drugs that modify the activity of that neurotransmitter. In the case of SSRIs, we have learned that serotonin plays a role in mood, anxiety, and impulsiveness—all symptoms that SSRIs help. Similarly, we know from the dopamine-modifying effects of stimulants like amphetamines and cocaine that this neurotransmitter regulates reward, pleasure, energy, as well as certain aspects of movement.

NEUROENDOCRINOLOGY

For several decades, psychiatric research approached the mind-brain complex by looking at hormonal responses to drugs. This field—how drugs affect hormones—is neuroendocrinology. And when we are dealing with mind-altering drugs, this is the field of psychoneuroendocrinology. Here is an example of how this model works. If amphetamine raises levels of the hormone adrenaline, we can suggest a role for adrenaline in the mood- and energy-elevating effects of amphetamine.

This was the approach I took in developing the DMT project, measuring multiple hormonal responses to the drug. Results would either support or refute the importance of specific hormones in mediating the DMT effect. And, if DMT increased one hormone but not another, we could work backward, proposing that DMT activated some serotonin receptors but not others.

Most psychedelics have potent neuroendocrine effects. For example, in our studies, we saw that DMT elevated blood levels of cortisol (a stress hormone), ACTH[13] (a pituitary hormone stimulating cortisol release), prolactin (involved with reproductive function and milk production), growth hormone, and beta-endorphin. Beta-endorphin is an opiate-like hormone and may be involved in some of DMT's especially pleasurable psychological

---

13. Adrenocorticotrophic hormone.

effects. We also saw extraordinary elevations of vasopressin after DMT administration. Vasopressin is similar to the prosocial bonding hormone oxytocin, and this might help explain the loving feelings our DMT volunteers sometimes felt after receiving the drug. In support of this theory, studies have recently shown that MDMA—an even more prosocial, bonding, "love drug"—stimulates the production of oxytocin. Oxytocin increases patients' trust in their therapists, and this might contribute to the robust positive effects that occur when combining MDMA with psychotherapy in PTSD and other disorders.

While neuroendocrine methods for studying psychedelics are less popular than the current interest in brain imaging, we ought to keep it in our toolbox as a unique approach to a fine-tuned analysis of the distinct receptors and hormones involved in the psychedelic effect. I say this because brain imaging studies are not yet able to reliably distinguish between different psychedelics—for example, between the classical compounds and MDMA—whereas neuroendocrine studies can.

BRAIN NETWORKS AND CONNECTIVITY

Advances in brain imaging technologies have dramatically increased our understanding of what happens after psychedelic drugs stimulate their relevant receptors. Such methods allow for more integrated models of psychedelic drug effects. The EEG—electroencephalogram—measures electrical activity on the brain's surface. Functional magnetic resonance imaging—fMRI—shows how active certain brain areas are by measuring their metabolism. PET—positron emission tomography—shows us where in the brain drugs go as well as their effects on metabolism. MEG—magnetoencephalography—measures magnetic fields that the brain produces. In addition, several technologies indicate how drugs affect blood flow to specific brain areas, an indirect measure of metabolic activity. In other words, more blood flows to metabolically active areas and less to metabolically quiet ones. These technologies have taught us the importance of brain networks and connectivity.

Networks within the brain consist of interconnected sites, or "hubs," which, acting in concert, regulate complex levels of mental function. Psychedelics affect the relationships between the brain's hubs—modifying connectivity within and among its several networks.

The default mode network (DMN) appears singularly important in relating psychedelics' subjective effects to changes in brain function. Its widely separated hubs regulate several "high-level" phenomena. These include the sense of self, orientation in space, attention, memory, anticipation, planning, meaningfulness, and how we relate to others. These functions are significantly more complex than those simply mediating, for example, vision. That is, they regulate the meaning and impact of visual perceptions, not simply their presence. We may even consider the DMN as the biological counterpart of the "ego"—the mental function that mediates between our "self" and the inner and outer worlds.

A term we frequently encounter in discussions of psychedelic effects on brain function is "entropy." Entropy refers to the degree of disorderliness, unpredictability, and randomness in any system at any point in time. Psychedelics increase whole brain entropy, and much of the data concerning brain networks and connectivity are reflections of this effect.

Increased brain entropy and the resulting changes in functional connectivity may translate into the psychedelic experience by altering the balance between "top-down" and "bottom-up" regulation of consciousness. Classical psychedelics—as well as ketamine, MDMA, and salvinorin A—all weaken connections within the DMN and between the DMN and "lower-level" networks and centers. Thus, there is a shift from "top-down" to "bottom-up" control and flow of information, as well as the specific centers that now exert more influence on each other. In other words, the DMN (the "top") no longer exerts as powerful an influence on lower-level networks (the "bottom"). These lower-level networks include those regulating sensory and emotional information. This allows previously DMN-suppressed/inhibited information to travel "upward" toward the "self." This self is now able to experience new, or newly significant, feelings, memories, and perceptions. Similarly, we know that LSD increases "response diversity" in the brain. Subjectively, this would correspond to psychedelics' ability to stimulate creativity and other processes that require novel mental associations.

There also are data pointing to a biological correspondence between the afterglow of the psychedelic drug experience and brain function. Some of the connectivity and entropy changes last for days to weeks after a single exposure to psilocybin. This has led to the notion of a "critical period" during which the mind-brain complex is especially susceptible to new input. Therapy, therefore, might be particularly effective during the days and weeks following a drug session, and not just during the acute intoxication.

PSYCHOPLASTOGENS

There is growing evidence for the importance of psychedelics' beneficial brain effects independent of their psychological ones. These effects are neurogenesis and neuroplasticity.

Neurogenesis refers to the growth of new neurons from stem cells in the brain. Stem cells are immature cells that may grow into any number of types, such as liver, heart, thyroid, as well as neurons. We now know that psychedelics stimulate the growth of new neurons. Neuroplasticity refers to the number and complexity of neural connections. We all have seen pictures of nerve cells with their intricate branching patterns. The more branches, the more connections are possible with other nerve cells. As in the case with neurogenesis, psychedelics also increase neuroplasticity.

These effects have led to a new term: "psychoplastogens."[14] While classical psychedelics produce psychoplastogenic effects, their mind-altering properties may not be necessary, at least in animal models. This is because non-psychedelic doses of psychedelics in lower animals are as psychoplastogenic as psychedelic doses. In addition, there are compounds closely related to psychedelics that are psychoplastogenic but not psychedelic, again in lower animals. Two examples of these latter compounds are modified versions of DMT and of ibogaine. Research using animal models of depression, drug abuse, and anxiety have demonstrated positive effects of non-psychedelic psychoplastogens.

In both cases—non-psychedelic doses and non-psychedelic drugs—a single exposure initiates psychoplastogenic effects within sixty to ninety minutes. This corresponds to the rapid remission of psychiatric symptoms with ketamine, psilocybin, and ayahuasca. These effects continue for weeks to a month. Of interest is that psilocybin's psychoplastogenic effects last longer than ketamine's. This may correspond to the need for repeating treatments with ketamine for depression at shorter intervals than is the case for psilocybin. These long-term psychoplastogenic effects may also underlie the afterglow phenomenon and the critical period for psychotherapy interventions.

These data are especially exciting. One reason is that the brains of those suffering from depression or schizophrenia demonstrate fewer neurons and less complexity of their interconnections. Psychoplastogens, therefore, may repair these deficits. Already, we have data showing that ayahuasca increases the thickness of cerebral cortex in humans. These findings are stimulating the development of human trials with psychedelics in

---

14. A more appropriate name might be "neuroplastogens," which would indicate that psychological effects are not necessary for these drugs' beneficial properties.

neurodegenerative diseases like ALS,[15] Parkinson's disease, and Alzheimer's dementia.

Test-tube studies show that nerve cells survive longer in conditions of low oxygen in the presence of DMT; and in the whole animal, DMT reduces the size of experimental stroke. Functional recovery from stroke also occurs more quickly in animals when DMT is present. These whole-animal effects appear at DMT doses that do not produce behavioral changes. Currently, we have very few options to treat either acute stroke, or to speed functional recovery. Imagine how important such therapies might prove in traumatic brain injury as well—a tragically common result of contact sports, accidents, combat, and domestic violence.

If psychoplastogenic effects are separable from psychedelic ones, such treatments will be more widely acceptable. This is because many patients would rather not have to undergo a profound mind-altering experience to obtain relief from their psychiatric and/or neurological conditions.

IMMUNE AND ANTI-INFLAMMATORY EFFECTS

We are just beginning to discover how the immune system responds to psychedelics. This is an especially promising avenue of future research because so many modern-day diseases result from abnormal immune and inflammatory function. These include autoimmune diseases, allergies, heart disease, dementia, gastrointestinal disorders, and cancer. Recent studies suggest that psychedelics are extraordinarily powerful anti-inflammatory drugs. As is the case with non-psychedelic psychoplastogens, some

---

15. Amyotrophic lateral sclerosis—"Lou Gehrig's disease"—where nerve cells enervating muscles die off, resulting in paralysis and early death. Stephen Hawking also suffered from ALS.

of these compounds do not appear psychedelic in lower animals or are effective at non-psychedelic doses.

CHAPTER 5

HOW PSYCHEDELICS WORK: THE MIND

It is within the mind that we are aware of the effects of psychedelic drugs. This is the world of subjectivity, inner experience, what we alone are conscious of. While not measurable in the same way as brain activity or hormonal responses, this is what is real to us, not the functional connectivity of the default mode network nor activation of serotonin receptors.

The previous chapter summarized the biological scientific data regarding psychedelic drug effects. These are precise numerical data. Powerful mathematical techniques demonstrate their "statistical significance." Nevertheless, they are less sensitive to what psychedelics are doing to us than is our subjective experience. For example, in our DMT work, volunteers' answers to questions on our rating scale—that is, their subjective experience—demonstrated differences between inactive saltwater placebo and an extremely low dose of drug. However, biological effects—such as elevated beta-endorphin blood levels—did not. But while subjective experience is more sensitive than biological data, our ability to agree on the nature of subjective experience is nowhere near as well developed. We lack consensus regarding vocabulary, concepts, and processes for the operation of the mind as an integrated whole.

Compared to brain science, we have innumerable theories of the mind— models for the normal mind, the diseased mind, and altered states of consciousness. Each possesses its own structures and mechanisms. We are thus dealing with "metaphysics" rather than a physical science—the physics, as it were, of subjective experience, things that only we have firsthand knowledge of, the "physics of the invisible." This situation provides fertile soil for any number of theories of the mind, since it is difficult to verify one or the other. In this context, I suggest not being misled by powerful statistical analyses of rating scale data that "prove" certain psychological theories. These rating scales attempt to capture elements of subjective experience, but how do we know if "sadness" or "happiness" means the same thing in different people? The expression "garbage in-garbage out" should exert a moderating influence on any such conclusions.

Among the theories of mind, the three I have studied most carefully are psychodynamic/psychoanalytic models, Buddhist ones, and those of medieval metaphysics.

FREUD'S PSYCHOANALYTIC/ PSYCHODYNAMIC MODEL

By "psychodynamic," I mean any model that teaches: "the child is the father to the man." We are the way we are because of how we were before. This emphasizes the importance of our interactions with people in our lives—especially in our early years. Those interactions combine with our physiological constitution, and thus we develop our unique personality. While we credit Freud for systematizing psychodynamic or "psychoanalytic" models, many have built upon his fundamental ideas. These are the schools of Jungian, cognitive behavioral, client-centered, motivational, and transpersonal therapies, among others.

Over one hundred years ago, Freud presented two complementary models for mental function. One consisted of the ego, superego, and id. These work together in allowing us to go about our daily lives. Do we work, follow societal norms, and experience the full range of emotions? As Freud once quipped about the meaning of life—if ego, superego, and id are working together well, we are able "to love and to work."

The id contains impulses and desires. If left to its own devices, the id's aggressive and sexual drives could wreak havoc. The superego contains family and cultural prohibitions that restrict the activity of the id. If life were all superego, it would be extraordinarily dull.[16] The ego mediates between these two competing forces. It is that with which we face the world: the people and objects in it, as well as our sense of ourselves. The ego is the "aware" aspect of the mind; it contains what is conscious, and it is where the competing interests of the id and superego play out.

Freud also proposed three levels of awareness, or consciousness. The conscious contains things that we are aware of moment to moment. For example, I am conscious of writing with a pen. Subconscious mental content is out of awareness but retrievable with a little effort, like what I had for breakfast this morning. It is where we find what we are trying to remember when something is on "the tip of the tongue." The unconscious, on the other hand, is inaccessible to awareness no matter how hard we try.

We know about the existence of the unconscious indirectly through its effects. These are feelings, thoughts, and behaviors that are inexplicable and may not serve us well, despite how hard we try to change them. In the psychodynamic model, clues regarding unconscious material emerge via dreams, slips of the tongue, humor, and—in psychotherapy—via the transference. This last concept refers to the relationship with one's therapist. Here, the goal is to use the relationship with the therapist to

---

16. An analogous model is that of the two "inclinations" in rabbinic Judaism—the "good" and the "evil" inclinations. With only a little irony, the saying goes that without the evil inclination, no one would get married, have children, make money, nor build a house. This points to the sexual, aggressive, and competitive properties of the id, and how they are necessary for many of the life experiences we all value, as well as continuation of our species.

clarify the nature of—and work to resolve—difficult relationships with important people in one's life.

These two models dovetail nicely. We—our ego—might be unconscious of the conflict between the id and the superego; for example, between a wish to hurt someone and the social forces preventing us. If these competing forces remain unconscious, we develop symptoms that represent an attempt to resolve the conflict. Say, if we have an unconscious wish to hurt our boss, the "neurotic" solution might be to get a migraine every time our boss wants to see us, rather than feel the rage behind the wish to harm him or her. However, these kinds of "solutions" are unsatisfactory because they cause distress and interfere with our lives.

We can propose that psychedelics modify the activities of either or both of these models' components. They may make more porous the barrier between the unconscious and conscious, whereby we become aware of previously unconscious memories or feelings. Feeling buried emotions now, in the present, and problem-solving our current circumstances using more mature and less rigid tools, helps the ego try innovative solutions. We then feel less burdened by vague, unidentifiable, unpleasant emotions or self-defeating behavior.

Psychedelics also might stimulate the production of visual symbols of conflicts or wishes—like dream images. One of our DMT volunteers saw herself travel through space to the Taj Mahal, and the beauty and opulence of the architecture stirred powerful, ecstatic feelings in her. In her daily life, she was living with a controlling, austere man who frowned upon pleasure, so a reasonable interpretation of her vision was that it represented fulfillment of wishes that she normally had to keep out of consciousness.

In addition, psychedelics may magnify the transference—feelings, thoughts, and associations regarding the psychedelic psychotherapist, or anyone of importance in the "setting." The magnification of the transference may shed light on how we relate to other important people in our lives.

Any or all of these processes, if successful, make us freer to consider new ways of being in the world and with ourselves. In other words, psychedelics amplify and magnify the ingredients of successful psychotherapy.[17]

Harkening back to the biological models I discussed in the previous chapter, there is a correspondence between brain entropy and functional connectivity with Freudian psychology. The ego—the sense of self that mediates our interactions with the inner and outer worlds—corresponds to the default mode network. Increasing brain entropy and connectivity among parts of the brain that are normally not well connected allows for the emergence of subconscious and especially unconscious material that the default mode network can now incorporate. Recollection of buried memories, new ideas, beliefs, resolution of emotional conflicts, and more adaptable courses of action may result. The mind becomes less rigid and more flexible.

BUDDHIST ABHIDHARMA PSYCHOLOGY

Another model I have carefully studied is Buddhist psychology, or Abhidharma.[18] I first learned about this Eastern system in the early 1970s. Later, in 1976, I spent a summer with a group of mental health professionals studying under a Tibetan Buddhist lama who taught us how to apply Abhidharma tools to our meditation.

---

17. How psychotherapy works, on the other hand, is mysterious in its own right. One of my supervisors during my psychiatry residency was a highly respected psychoanalyst who taught at the San Francisco Psychoanalytic Institute. One day, I asked him how he thought psychotherapy worked. In all seriousness (or in jest—I never really found out), he replied, "I think it's like monkeys picking lice off of each other's backs."

18. There are three "baskets" comprising Buddhist teachings. The *Sutras*, discourses that the Buddha and his disciples gave on assorted topics; Vinaya, the rules of the monastic community; and Abhidharma, Buddhist psychology.

Abhidharma is a phenomenological approach to the mind and states of consciousness; in particular, altered states of consciousness that diverse types of meditation produce. By "phenomenological," I mean isolating the components of subjective experience without adding any additional interpretations or explanations. It is "the facts and just the facts." Rather than calling something a "near-death experience," the phenomenological approach would describe the characteristics of that state—for example, a white light, great peace, flying through space, the loss of a sense of time, etc.

The Abhidharma's model of mind consists of five independent and interactive functions working together in such a way as to give the impression of "ongoing experience." These are body awareness, feeling and emotion, thoughts and thought processes, perception, and volition or sense of self. These are like the categories of mental function that all medical students learn to assess when interviewing psychiatric patients during their psychiatry rotation. In developing our scale, I combined these two approaches—clinical psychiatry and Buddhist psychology—and included questions tapping each Abhidharma/"mental status" category. In the case of "emotions/feeling," for example, the Hallucinogen Rating Scale (HRS) asked about how "safe," "fearful," "peaceful," or "anxious" the individual felt during their experience. We then tallied these responses to calculate an "emotion" score.

Scores on the HRS provide a phenomenological profile of a drug effect.[19] One can say, for example, that DMT is more "perceptual" than MDMA, which might instead lean more heavily toward "emotional."

We can use the Buddhist model to understand how psychedelics might produce benefit in those who take them. Buddhism emphasizes the realization of the illusory nature of everyday existence. There is fundamentally no "self" that experiences the unhappiness that

---

19. In fact, it can provide a profile of any altered state of consciousness.

accompanies much of daily life. All phenomena are "empty" of essential existence. Instead, reality consists of an endless arising, existing, and passing away of phenomena. If psychedelics, therefore, could help one attain that knowledge, suffering will automatically diminish because it is a more truthful assessment of reality. Research has demonstrated improved results of meditation in those who have taken psilocybin during a Buddhist retreat, so there are data supporting this notion.

It is important to remember that the millennia-old teachings of Buddhism provide a cognitive verbal platform for understanding, integrating, and applying these altered states of consciousness. I believe these cognitive models also are applicable to altered states that come about through psychedelics. Without concrete time-tested guidelines, the nonverbal, mostly self-centered, intuitive nature of these experiences—meditative or psychedelic—lends itself to "making it up as you go along." Solid intellectual, moral, and ethical grounding makes it less likely that one overlays the experience of "emptiness," for example, with whatever misguided philosophies they choose.

MEDIEVAL METAPHYSICS

I wish to introduce a model dating back to the Greek philosopher-scientist Aristotle that I believe is useful in understanding both the psychological and spiritual effects of psychedelic drugs. In this, I use the version that the medieval Jewish philosophers developed, especially that of Maimonides—a rabbi, philosopher, and physician who lived in Egypt in the 1200s. I am the first to admit the idiosyncratic nature of this model, but please bear with me, and I think you will see why I find it attractive.

Aristotle divided the mind into two "faculties," or functions. One is the rational faculty, or intellect. The other is the imaginative faculty, or imagination.

The rational faculty is the location in the mind for abstractions, thoughts, beliefs, and concepts. Things that have no discernible form. That is, we do not see an idea, we think it. The rational faculty is where we experience concepts, remember them, and combine them in new ways. Mathematics is a good example of the contents and operations of the rational faculty. For the medievalists, nonphysical thoughts provided a link between our minds and a nonphysical God. The rational faculty is what distinguishes humans from "beasts." It is the manifestation of our spiritual nature.

The imaginative faculty is the location of everything else. It contains "physical" information, such as sensations, body awareness, and emotions. As such, the philosophers believed that the imaginative faculty was physical, biological, something that we share with lower animals. The "imagination" in this system differs from the common definition of "imaginary," "unreal," "make-believe," and the like. Instead, it is simply the location of everything nonabstract that exists in our minds. It is where we experience nonabstract contents, remember them, and create novel combinations such as works of art.

The medievalists proposed that the imaginative faculty, being biological in nature, was not especially amenable to change. They knew of no way to increase the function of the imagination. As they located it in the brain, this meant that the brain constrained the function of the imagination. The best one could do was to not degrade its function through an unhealthy lifestyle. The rational faculty, on the other hand, was amenable to growth and development through study and living a virtuous life. That virtuous life would also help maintain the health of the brain.

For Maimonides, the attainment of prophecy—the highest possible spiritual experience in the Hebrew biblical tradition—occurred with the "perfection" of the imagination and intellect working in concert. This was quite rare because of how infrequently one encountered a "perfected" brain, as well as the rigors of study and morality necessary to perfect the intellect.

In the case of the prophet, the perfection of the intellect and the imagination resulted in heightened receptivity to externally existent divine information. It was not a case of "influencing God" to communicate with the prophet. Rather, the state of the prophet made him/her more capable of receiving divine influence that was constantly everywhere.

Maimonides's model proposes that divine influence stimulated the imagination from outside the person. The imagination then converted this influence into things one could perceive: visions, voices, feelings, and other "bodily" contents. Because of the divine source of the imagination's contents, those contents contained divine information. A perfected imagination would allow for more clear and discernible contents than those one perceived via a weak, corrupted imagination.

Then, a perfected intellect would extract information from the perfectly perceived, divinely generated contents of the imagination. This information is now verbal, conceptual, abstract. A perfected intellect is also able to effectively communicate that information verbally to others. There are hundreds of examples of this process in the Hebrew Bible's account of prophetic experience.[20]

Here is how I see psychedelics fitting into this model. Up until now, we have been unable to significantly modify the biological imagination. We are born with a more or less well-developed brain. Our senses are only so sharp, our emotions only so refined. Psychedelics, however, may be a route to stimulating the imagination.

During my DMT work, I was impressed by how the psychedelic experience was much more "imaginative" than "intellectual." Volunteers could describe in extraordinary detail the feelings, visions, emotions, and bodily properties of the experience. However, the quantity and novelty of the cognitive

---

20. By prophetic experience, I mean any altered state of consciousness in which a human and the divine interact in the Hebrew Bible. This extends the definition from simply "prediction" or "foretelling."

contents were relatively meager. The experiences simply confirmed or extended volunteers' preexisting beliefs, or helped clarify personal problems, enhancing their meaning, imbuing them with a greater sense of truth and reality. I believe this is the result of a stimulated imagination. How one determines what is real ultimately relates to "how it feels." It is a feeling, not a rational deduction. And feeling is in the domain of the imagination.

Thus, it seems as if DMT and other psychedelics stimulate the imagination more than the intellect. In this, they provide a tool to strengthen the imagination in a way that was not available to the medievalists.

There are two ways in which a "stimulated imagination" may impart new information to someone in the psychedelic state. One is the aforementioned heightened receptivity or sensitivity to spiritual information that surrounds us at all times. This is the basis of my "theoneurological" model of spiritual experience, an alternative to the top-down model of "neurotheology." Neurotheology, the reigning model for the biology of spiritual experience, treats such experiences from a bottom-up perspective. The brain generates the impression of communicating with the divine, perhaps through the release of endogenous DMT through the activation of a brain reflex brought about by prayer. The top-down model, theoneurology, proposes that the world of spirit communicates with us through the brain. Endogenous DMT, from this perspective, allows formless divine information to become perceptible.

The better developed one's intellect, the more capable one is in deciphering the contents of the stimulated imagination. This is where I see the role of the intellect—which our "set" contains—in determining what we learn from any psychedelic experience. On one hand, a trip may be primarily "imaginative"—an aesthetic experience—fun, exciting, interesting, and novel. Or it may be the source of more practical and enduring information if one possesses the intention, vocabulary, and similar tools to mine the newly rich imaginative contents.

I hope this metaphysical approach helps underscore an important point, one that is fundamental in determining the outcome of any psychedelic experience. The more tools you have at your disposal to process what the drug shows you, the more you will get out of it. No matter the source of the imaginative contents—divine, extraterrestrial, or psychological—the better developed the intellect, the more information one can extract from them.

A NOTE ON THE BEINGS

DMT, salvinorin A, and ketamine often disclose the presence of "beings." These are autonomous figures that appear in our visions. They may take any number of forms: human or humanoid, animal, plant, machine, or insect. They possess power, intelligence, and will. They interact and communicate with us more or less effectively using telepathy and/or nonverbal methods. In my DMT research, the volunteers and I discussed the beings at great length. Who or what are they? Where do they reside? How does one relate to them?

Early on in my studies, I needed to engage in a thought experiment in order to maintain open channels of communication with my volunteers. This involved taking at face value the "more real than real" nature of the DMT world, including its inhabitants—the beings. Otherwise, if I reacted to volunteers' accounts by interpreting their experiences as other than their face value—by considering them as drug-induced hallucinations or unconscious Freudian conflicts that are now conscious—they were less inclined to share some of the most interesting aspects of their experiences. After wrapping up my studies, I explored various models that could explain the reality-basis of the beings and their world.

I looked at several models and freely speculated as to their relevance in *DMT: The Spirit Molecule*. While anything is possible, I admit to the impossibility of solving this puzzle—the location of the DMT world and those who seem to exist there. The only explanation I can give is generic and returns to the definition of "psychedelic." These substances make visible the previously invisible.

Using the metaphysicians' system, we can point to the "imagination" as the location of the beings. This is where we perceive them: their appearance, what we hear, how we feel around them both physically and emotionally. At the same time, they contain information. We can learn something from them. This information is "clothed" in a manner that we can perceive. However, it is impossible to determine if this information comes from within or outside of us. All we can say with certainty is that it was previously invisible. The task of extracting information from the beings, as with any other "imaginative" content, is the job of the intellect, the rational faculty.

SUBJECTIVE EXPERIENCE AND OUTCOME

When scientists believe that a particular type of psychedelic experience causes benefit, they develop a rating scale that measures that experience. Upon finding correlations between that experience and outcome, they point to its attainment in explaining how psychedelics work.

However, it may be that any number of other experiences correlate just as strongly with outcome. For example, a recent study demonstrated an association between scores on the Mystical Experience Questionnaire (MEQ) and decreased alcohol consumption in alcoholics. The MEQ is a rating scale that quantifies elements of the mystical-unitive state and determines if one's "mystical experience" is "complete" or "incomplete." However, the correlation between a generic measure of drug-effect intensity was also strong. That is, the intensity of the experience, not its specific quality, was important.

Here is another example. Psychiatric researchers who used LSD to treat alcoholics in Saskatchewan believed that LSD caused a time-limited case of the DTs, or delirium tremens. Delirium tremens is a clinical syndrome in which withdrawing alcoholics undergo a nightmarish descent into extraordinary physical and mental anguish. Since many alcoholics stop drinking after the DTs, this model suggested that to the extent that DT-like symptoms occurred on LSD, alcohol consumption would cease. And this is what they found. Therefore, might scores on a "DT rating scale" demonstrate the same correlations with outcome as those measured by the MEQ? Similarly, would we see an association between improvement in treatment-resistant depression or pain with high "DT scores" as with scores on the "Ego Dissolution Scale"?

People take and/or give psychedelics within the set and setting of a particular model. If researchers and subjects believe that the DTs or mystical experiences are curative, and if rating scales measure the attainment of the state, it is likely that the attainment of that state will relate to outcome. That is, the drug effect—and the rating scale that establishes its attainment—confirms the model.

When we believe that attaining a particular subjective experience is "how psychedelics work," we may be veering dangerously close to "magical thinking." That is, the belief that "all you need to do is reach this state and it doesn't matter what your problems are. They will magically succumb to the effect of the state."[21]

---

21. This is why the psychedelic psychotherapy research team at the University of Maryland failed to receive a renewal grant from the National Institutes of Health in the early 1970s. Eberhardt Uhlenhuth was one of my mentors in New Mexico and was on the site visit determining whether to continue funding their work. According to Dr. Uhlenhuth, the Baltimore research team—which included William Richards, now the lead psychedelic psychotherapist at Johns Hopkins—"had gotten religion." They were no longer interested in *how* psychedelics worked. Rather, they knew it was through the attainment of a mystical experience. It was now only a matter of applying that state to any number of conditions.

You cannot similarly argue that objective brain-function changes that occur in the mystical or any other specific state prove that such states are indeed how "psychedelics work." This is because those brain changes may simply reflect the operation of a nonspecific brain response to the psychedelic experience—for example, its intensity. That intensity may be the critical factor more than the attainment of any specific mental state.

While many of the characteristics of a mystical experience and its aftereffects appear to be beneficial, it is important to remain discerning. Increased "acceptance," "openness," and "compassion" accompanying such an experience may not always be a good thing. Do we really want to be more accepting of violent racist ideology and behavior? Some people do, and we therefore see psychedelics' use in such settings. Do we want to be more compassionate to those who wish to hurt us or our loved ones? Likewise, the nonverbal "ineffable" properties of the drug-induced mystical state are open to abuse and manipulation. That is, if the information content of such experiences is a blank slate, one may fall prey to the influence of false, if not frankly malignant, beliefs and influences.

CHAPTER 6

PSYCHEDELICS, PANACEAS, PLACEBOS, AND PSYCHOPLASTOGENS

This chapter takes us into speculative territory, so before digging into it, I want to state what I am proposing. Please keep in mind these are theoretical considerations, not established facts. However, I believe they provide promising directions for future research into how psychedelics work.

This hypothesis suggests that the panacea-like properties of psychedelics are due to their biological effects enhancing the placebo response. This they do through their psychoplastogenic properties—growing new nerve cells and increasing the complexity of their connections. These psychoplastogenic mechanisms operate even without a psychedelic experience. Nevertheless, with or without a psychedelic experience, set and setting remain crucial in determining the outcome of any administration of a "psychedelic" drug.

Controlled clinical trials with psychedelics indicate that they are effective treatments for depression, alcoholism, tobacco and opiate dependence, obsessive-compulsive disorder, PTSD, pain, autism, anxiety, and end-of-life despair. They also improve meditation, enhance the commitment of clerics to their pastoral mission, and modify one's personality to become more open, flexible, accepting, and compassionate. Studies originating outside of the research laboratory suggest that psychedelics increase nature appreciation and domestic conviviality; foster progressive politics; change metaphysical beliefs; and reduce prisoner recidivism, the severity of eating disorders and headache, and symptoms of fibromyalgia. They may even be useful for neurodegenerative diseases like dementia, stroke, traumatic brain injury, Parkinson's disease, and ALS. We also know that neo-Nazi and other radical groups take psychedelics to strengthen their beliefs, and that Charles Manson administered LSD to his followers to cement their status as serial killers.

PANACEA AND PLACEBO

A panacea—from the Latin "all-healing" or "cure-all"—is a solution or remedy for all difficulties or diseases. In medical/psychological contexts, a panacea may be a completely inert substance like a sugar pill. This is the classic "placebo." Or it may have biological effects that likewise help innumerable disorders. This is what we call an active placebo. When the biologically active Prozac first came out, people hailed it as a panacea. Its serotonin reuptake inhibiting effects led to theories regarding how "correcting serotonin deficiency" explained its broad efficacy. Similarly, I believe that psychedelics' biological effects also underlie their heal-all properties.

Placebo is Latin for "I shall please" or "I shall be pleasing." Placebos may be inert or active biologically. We now know that even "inert" placebos like a sugar pill have measurable objective biological effects. These include immune, inflammatory, hormonal, and functional brain changes. For example, endorphins—the body's own pain-reducing opioid hormones—mediate placebo analgesia. We know this because the opiate/endorphin-blocking drug naloxone inhibits placebo analgesia.

The placebo effect is the extent to which the response we see to a treatment is greater or otherwise different from what we might expect from that treatment alone. The placebo effect plays a role in everyday medical practice: a prescriber encourages a positive response to a heart medication, asthma inhaler, even chemotherapy for cancer. They will say, "I believe this will help you and I expect it to." In the world of psychiatry, we see the same mechanisms at work when combining psychotherapy with antidepressants. The two together work better than either alone. This is an example of how the setting—in this case, the supportive and encouraging psychotherapeutic context—improves the effect of a biologically active treatment.

A functional definition of the placebo effect is the recruitment of the mind-brain complex's innate psychological and biological mechanisms of change. When the treatment possesses biological effects, the placebo contribution is additive, making that treatment more effective.

This definition does not assume that recruiting those innate mechanisms results only in healing. The activation of innate biological and psychological change processes may result in negative outcomes, too. The nocebo response describes how negative expectations about a prognosis or treatment make their occurrence more likely. The specific effects of placebo are dependent upon set and setting; that is, what those receiving and those providing any intervention wish and expect to see.

A CLOSER LOOK AT SET AND SETTING

Set refers to who we are at the time of our psychedelic drug experience. Mental and physical health play key roles. For this chapter's purposes, I wish to emphasize specific elements of set. These are selection bias, expectancy, suggestibility, and hypnotizability.

Selection bias influences who decides to take a psychedelic drug in the first place. People take psychedelics—within or outside a research setting—because of their interest in them. Depressed patients volunteering for a psilocybin-treatment study believe that psilocybin may improve their mood. Therefore, they are fundamentally different from those who do not believe this. Those who take ayahuasca at Latin American retreat centers also believe it will be of benefit. These are expectations of particular outcomes. People without those expectations will not self-select to participate in such activities, and they may even respond to psilocybin or ayahuasca differently from those with expectations.

Expectancy is a state of thinking or hoping that something will happen or be the case. What someone is expecting may be either positive or negative.

Suggestibility is the quality of being inclined to believe certain things, and to act on the suggestions of others. Someone who is more suggestible is also more likely to be hypnotizable; that is, susceptible to hypnosis. There is also the phenomenon of "auto-suggestion," where one suggests certain things to themself. This is the idea behind self-affirmations one practices in an altered state like meditation or deep relaxation, both of which may increase suggestibility.

In addition to the physical environment, setting includes the set of those around you. Those giving you psychedelics have certain expectations as to what the drugs will do and suggest that you will experience those effects. They also will suggest how to attain them when you are in the altered state. "Do this and that will happen." These are suggestions. One way to make a desired outcome more likely is through increasing suggestibility. And hypnosis does just that. So do psychedelics.

Hypnosis is an enhanced capacity to respond to suggestion. Often, this enhanced capacity comes about through an altered state of consciousness—the "trance." The more suggestible someone is, the more susceptible they are to hypnosis. Some refer to hypnosis as "placebo without deception." In hypnosis, one knows that they are receiving a suggestion that something will happen. When they believe they are receiving a pharmacologically active substance—say, a painkiller—the suggestion of effect positively influences the result—pain relief. The "trance"—or altered state of consciousness—making suggestibility more effective comes about through the trappings associated with the clinical setting. They are "entranced" by the white-coated doctor with an authoritative air and diplomas on the walls, friendly yet crisply efficient nurses, and the smell of the waiting room. Their belief about the pill is part of the "set." The accoutrements and expectations that the clinical environment comprise are the "setting."

The relationships among placebo, hypnosis, suggestibility, and expectancy are complex and multidirectional. Greater expectation of response improves the rate of response. Those with high expectations may be more innately suggestible. These differences in suggestibility may impact the role of expectation; in other words, the more suggestible someone is, the greater their expectation of effect. Increased suggestibility may therefore predict greater placebo response. That is, these mechanisms work together to produce an end result: enhanced placebo response—the observed outcome is greater than that expected from the treatment itself.

A key element in the placebo response is that it occurs outside of awareness—it is unconscious. There are no subjective correlates of an activated placebo response. We may see the results of this activation—say, pain relief—but we do not see, hear, smell, or experience anything conscious during placebo's operation.

PSYCHEDELICS AND THE PLACEBO EFFECT

How, then, do psychedelics fit into our discussion of hypnosis, expectancy, suggestibility, panacea, and placebo?

Psychedelic drugs are unrivaled in their ability to produce any number of effects—those that the person who takes them desires as well the desires of those who administer them But psychedelics are not inert placebos acting solely through hypnosis or enhanced suggestibility. They also have powerful biological effects. These effects interact with set and setting.[22] Therefore, one might consider psychedelics to magnify the placebo response through their biological properties.

Experiments in the 1960s showed that hypnosis plus LSD caused a more intense altered state than either LSD or hypnosis alone. In this case, the suggestion was to experience a "psychedelic" altered state. LSD magnified the effects of hypnosis/suggestion, and hypnosis/suggestion magnified the effects of LSD. These findings led to the development of "hypnodelic therapy."

More recent data also demonstrate that LSD increases suggestibility. In addition, subjects who take an inert placebo when in the company of people pretending to be intoxicated with a psychedelic drug experience psychedelic effects. These two parallel sets of modern-day data support the original 1960s studies: LSD increases suggestibility, and suggestion leads to a psychedelic experience.

However, psychedelics do not always produce the desired outcome. This may be because they do not always magnify the placebo response and/ or because the condition is not placebo-responsive. It also may be that placebo activation requires attaining a particular "psychedelic experience." As I suggest in the previous chapter, instead of any specific state mediating

---

22. This interplay among drug, set, setting, hypnosis, expectancy, and suggestibility helps explain why psychedelics were not especially effective brainwashing or programming tools. For psychedelics to "turn someone into an assassin," there must first be preexisting, more or less conscious, murderous/violent impulses in one's set. Without the proper set, it is unlikely that one can manipulate the setting so as to simply implant out of whole cloth a foreign set of beliefs. No one in any of the present-day psychedelic research studies has become a serial killer. Likewise, no one in Manson's group became a monk while a member of his group.

outcome, the key ingredient may be the intensity of the experience. By intensity, I mean a feeling of profound meaningfulness and significance. Statements such as "this is more real than real" or "this was the most significant experience of my life" capture the essence of the feeling that something momentous has taken place. Therefore, we can propose that the subjective correlate of psychedelic activation of an enhanced placebo-response is a state of consciousness reaching a critical threshold of intensity.

We can address these questions experimentally. For example, do more suggestible people respond more robustly to psychedelic-assisted treatments? Do conditions that are more placebo responsive like allergies improve more than those that are not, like cancer?

NON-PSYCHEDELIC PSYCHOPLASTOGENIC PSYCHEDELICS

The discovery of psychoplastogens and their potential benefits in psychiatric disorders has added a fascinating wrinkle into this discussion. They raise the possibility that no subjective experience is necessary for psychedelics to exert their therapeutic actions.

Non-psychedelic doses of psychedelics like DMT, psilocybin, and ketamine increase neurogenesis—the growth of new neurons in the brain. They also increase neuroplasticity—the number and complexity of connections among neurons. In animals, laboratory-modified versions of DMT and ibogaine are psychoplastogenic but not psychedelic. These non-psychedelic psychoplastogens also show effectiveness in lower animal models of anxiety, depression, and addiction.

In humans, there also exists a relationship between psychoplastogenic and antidepressant effects. Brain cell loss and decreased connectivity occur in certain psychiatric conditions. It therefore is reasonable to believe that stimulating neurogenesis and neuroplasticity would be beneficial in these disorders. I have already referred to how long-term ayahuasca use in humans increases the thickness of certain areas of the cerebral cortex. Also in humans, psychedelics' antidepressant effects occur within the same time span—sixty to ninety minutes—in which we see increases in neuroplasticity in animal models. In addition, these effects continue over time—a couple of weeks to a month—and may correspond in humans to the afterglow or "critical period" during which milder but real benefit continues to accrue after one's drug session. Remember, too, that this critical period is one in which the effects of psychotherapy may be especially powerful—that is, a time of enhanced suggestibility.

The development of non-psychedelic psychoplastogens severs the linkage between psychoplastogenic and psychedelic properties. While a sufficiently intense mental state may reflect the activation of the psychoplastogenic response, this same response may occur in the absence of a psychedelic experience.

Therapeutic responses to psychoplastogens do not require a psychedelic experience, at least in lower animals. If this were also true in humans, the therapeutic response would occur outside of conscious awareness.[23] The same is true for the placebo response—we are unconscious of its operation. Are the two phenomena related? That is, do psychoplastogenic effects underlie placebo ones? If they do, this may occur by increasing suggestibility and hypnotizability, mechanisms that contribute to the placebo response. This is a key question and we can answer it experimentally. That is, do non-psychedelic psychoplastogens increase suggestibility?

Like placebo, psychedelic or non-psychedelic psychoplastogenic effects are nonspecific. They both require direction, and that direction involves set and setting. The new connections among nerve cells are not random but

---

23. If these substances do induce an altered state, that state would not be psychedelic.

will reflect the biopsychosocial circumstances in which they take place. For example, the new, more complex connections that develop while watching violent pornography would develop differently from those occurring while meditating in the forest.

Even without psychedelic effects, psychotherapy and other methods to direct these compounds' psychoplastogenic properties will most likely yield more benefit than prescribing them alone. It will be fascinating to determine if psychotherapy in combination with psychedelic psychoplastogens is more effective than psychotherapy in combination with non-psychedelic ones. If not, then non-psychedelic psychoplastogens might simply turn out to be like regular antidepressants—effective on their own, but probably not as effective as when one is also in psychotherapy. At the very least, the acceptability and practicality of non-psychedelic compounds will be greater for the public than those requiring the rigors of a highly altered state.

When using psychoplastogens in solely neurological conditions such as dementia or stroke, similar considerations for optimizing the setting also are important. The regeneration of damaged brain areas will be most effective in combination with physical therapy and other rehabilitative procedures that optimally direct that regeneration.

But how about those who wish to experience a psychedelic effect? This situation sits at the other end of the spectrum whose opposite pole is using non-psychedelic psychoplastogens for neurological conditions. Pleasure, recreation, and enhancement of aesthetic experience are valid reasons to take a psychedelic drug and are the most popular reasons for doing so.

It is in the middle of this spectrum, in the case of psychiatric and wellness settings, that the balance between psychedelic and non-psychedelic psychoplastogenic effects is most relevant. Here, I believe we will find that non-psychedelic psychoplastogens may be effective on their own, but they will be more so when combined with psychotherapy, meditation, and other methods that take advantage of expectancy and suggestibility.

If so, so what?

What are the practical consequences of this proposal—that psychedelics magnify the placebo response via their psychoplastogenic effects? This hypothesis provides a functional link between the role of set and setting and biology. It objectifies the subjective reality of how set and setting determine the outcome of any individual drug experience. The relationship between mind and body becomes ever more undeniable.

PART III

THE PSYCHEDELIC DRUGS

CHAPTER 7

CLASSICAL PSYCHEDELICS

These are the compounds that most of us think of when we hear the term "psychedelic drug." We know the most about them, and they have the longest history of use both indigenously and in the modern West. They include natural substances that occur in the plant and animal kingdom: mescaline in peyote and San Pedro cacti, psilocybin in "magic" mushrooms, DMT in a multitude of plants and animals, ibogaine in the iboga plant, and 5-methoxy-DMT in the venom of the Sonoran Desert toad. LSD is synthetic but is a derivative of a naturally occurring fungus that grows on domestic grains.

MESCALINE, PEYOTE, AND SAN PEDRO

Indigenous use of the mescaline-containing peyote cactus extends further back into history than most any other botanical psychedelic. The discovery of mescaline and its psychoactive effects marks the beginning of Western scientific interest in psychedelic drugs.

HISTORY

Mescaline-containing peyote and San Pedro cacti have played a role in Western hemisphere Indigenous social, healing, and religious spheres for millennia. Traditional names for the peyote cactus include *hikuri* and *hikuli*. Indigenous populations that we identify with peyote's use are the Huichol and Tarahumara of Mexico. Peyote's botanical name is *Lophophora williamsii*. Its use was prominent among the Aztecs and in pre-Aztec rituals that may extend back five thousand years.

San Pedro's use centered in and around modern-day Peru, and may be over three thousand years old. There are several species of psychoactive San Pedro cacti, all belonging to the genus *Trichocereus* (alternatively, *Echinopsis*). Common species are *T. pachanoi* and *T. peruvianus*. Traditional names include *huachuma* and *wachuma*.

Indigenous use of peyote migrated northward and combined with Christianity to become the Native American Church (NAC) in the late 1800s. This is the largest Native American religion, claims nearly a quarter-million adherents, and extends up to the Canadian prairies of Saskatchewan. Other Native American peyote-using religious groups are free of Christian influence.

The German pharmacologist Louis Lewin first described the psychedelic effects of peyote in the 1880s. He discusses peyote in his 1924 book *Phantastica*. Mescaline saw use in the early days of psychedelic research, beginning in the 1920s. These were studies that employed mescaline to produce a "model psychosis." Therapists also used it as a psychotherapeutic aid. Other research engaged in what we would now call "psychophysiology" studies; for example, cataloging the types of visual phenomena that the drug produced in normal volunteers. In addition, Canadian researchers' interest in model psychoses led to biochemical theories of schizophrenia, some of which continue to inform contemporary research.

Mescaline's long duration of action—up to twelve hours—was unwieldy in the clinical research setting, and nausea and vomiting were not uncommon. Thus, it never quite captured the scientific and popular attention that LSD did later. The latter compound's much greater potency, and its appearance at the dawn of modern psychopharmacology, worked to its advantage and relegated mescaline to the psychedelic social and research backwoods. However, as Indigenous use of psychedelics is increasingly relevant, commercial, social, and academic interest in mescaline is greater now than it has been in many years.

Aldous Huxley's 1954 book, *The Doors of Perception*, is an articulate account of the aesthetic, spiritual, and intellectual effects of mescaline in this highly educated philosopher. Perhaps more than any other, this book stimulated interest in psychedelics among artists, academics, and the youth culture.

BOTANY

Peyote is a slow-growing, spineless, button-shaped cactus that may take fifteen to twenty years to reach maturity. Its native habitat is northern Mexico and southwest Texas, where it is now an endangered species because of overharvesting. The cactus may attain a diameter of up to seven inches and a height of up to three inches. San Pedro, on the other hand, is a fast-growing columnar cactus that may attain heights of up to twenty feet. San Pedro has a wide distribution in Central and South America and grows easily in cultivation.

CHEMISTRY/PHARMACOLOGY

Arthur Heffter, a German chemist, isolated mescaline from peyote in the 1890s and identified it as peyote's primary psychoactive component. The Viennese chemist Ernst Späth synthesized mescaline in 1919.

Mescaline is a phenethylamine. Therefore, it is unique among the classical compounds, the remainder of which are tryptamines.[24] However, its pharmacology is similar—affecting primarily postsynaptic serotonin receptors, in particular the 5-HT2A.

Alexander Shulgin used mescaline as the starting point for hundreds of novel phenethylamines with more or less psychedelic properties. These include DOM, DOET, DOB, DOI, and 2C-B, some of which either have seen or are seeing use in research and/or in the psychedelic underground.

DOSE AND ROUTE OF ADMINISTRATION

A psychedelic oral dose—the preferred route—of pure mescaline is between 300–600 mg.

People consume peyote fresh or dried. When dried, one may either eat dried buttons or powdered cactus, or drink a peyote tea. Depending on the concentration of mescaline in the dried peyote, one may need between 30–150 g of buttons, or four to twelve average-sized ones. For San Pedro, a usual dose of fresh cactus is about a one-foot section of a two- to three-inch diameter piece. There is more mescaline in the green skin of San Pedro than other parts of the plant. One may powder the dried skin or boil a blended slurry of the whole plant.[25] With both San Pedro and peyote, concentrations of mescaline can differ significantly, which may require more or less plant material for an effective dose.

EFFECTS AND SIDE EFFECTS

Effects of pure oral mescaline begin within thirty to sixty minutes, while onset of cactus effects may be even longer, two to four hours. Thus, one must be careful not to prematurely take additional plant material until

---

24. Other phenethylamines include MDMA and the non-psychedelic amphetamines and methamphetamines.

25. To avoid nausea and vomiting from the slurry, some people administer it as an enema.

enough time has passed to make certain it is safe to do so. Effects may last up to twelve to fourteen hours. Claims of qualitative differences between mescaline and other classical drugs are difficult to confirm.

Mescaline may possess more inherently unpleasant gastrointestinal side effects than other classical drugs. In addition, mescaline-containing cacti are quite bitter and have other compounds with noxious gastrointestinal effects. These additional considerations increase the likelihood of nausea, vomiting, and occasionally, diarrhea with either peyote or San Pedro.

LEGAL

The Controlled Substances Act lists mescaline as a Schedule I drug. It is illegal to use, possess, distribute, manufacture, or sell. However, the American Religious Freedom Restoration Act of 1993 reaffirmed the right of Indigenous religious groups to use peyote in their rituals.

Some peyote churches exclude non-Natives, while others allow all races. In addition, some states forbid non-Native participation in NAC ceremonies. With these caveats, religious use of peyote by the NAC is legal in the US. Some states also allow "religious use" of peyote outside of the NAC. The peyote plant is not illegal to possess in the US if one does not intend to use it for psychedelic effects. Exceptions exist in other countries—for example, in France and Brazil—where the plant itself is illegal. Because the peyote cactus is endangered, its collection is prohibited except for purposes of traditional use by Indigenous groups.

San Pedro is legal for gardening purposes, but not for use as a psychedelic. Nevertheless, some countries outlaw San Pedro; for example, Switzerland. Collecting San Pedro in the wild is not illegal.

LSD

The discovery and widespread use of LSD (lysergic acid diethylamide, or "acid") unleashed powerful scientific and social forces in the 1950s and 1960s. Scientific, in that the drug firmly established the legitimacy and power of the new discipline of psychopharmacology—how brain chemistry affects subjective experience, both normal and abnormal. Socially, in its power to heighten the intensity of countercultural impulses previously latent in the post-World War II West. These impulses found their outlet in massive protest movements against a host of societal ills.

HISTORY

Ergot and other fungi that grow on domesticated grains and other grasses produce psychoactive LSD-like compounds, such as lysergic acid amide (LSA, or ergine). This compound also appears in the seeds of several vines, including Hawaiian baby woodrose and certain morning glories. The use of LSA-containing botanicals extends thousands of years into antiquity, both in the Americas and Greece. The Aztecs utilized the seeds of the vine *ololiuqui* (*Ipomoea corymbosa*) for religious and shamanic purposes, and its use in Mesoamerica continues. Participants in the Greek Eleusinian Mysteries drank an ergot-containing drink called *kykeon* in rituals that ended in the 400s CE.

LSD does not occur in nature. Albert Hofmann synthesized it in 1938 while working at Sandoz Pharmaceuticals. It was one of a series of compounds he developed to stimulate respiratory and cardiovascular function without causing uterine contraction side effects. He inadvertently discovered its psychedelic effects five years later, probably by absorbing it through his skin. This discovery set off a flurry of basic and clinical scientific research that continues to this day.

LSD's remarkable potency—orally active at millionths of a gram—captured the scientific and public imagination to a much greater extent than did the less potent and more side-effect–prone mescaline. In addition, the similarity between LSD's pharmacology and chemistry and that of the recently discovered serotonin—the first known neurotransmitter—ushered in the new science of psychopharmacology: how drugs affect the mind.

During the first wave of interest in psychedelics, scientists studied LSD's effects across a dizzying scientific landscape. These included its use as a treatment—with or without additional individual or group psychotherapy—for depression, autism, alcohol and heroin addiction, schizophrenia, end-of-life despair, sociopathy, and pain. In addition, studies investigated its ability to enhance empathy in clinicians treating psychotic patients. Finally, its power to provide insight into the serotonin system led to the development of two new families of psychopharmacological agents: the SSRI antidepressants and the second-generation antipsychotics like risperidone and olanzapine.

CHEMISTRY/PHARMACOLOGY

LSD's pharmacology is typical of the other classical psychedelics; that is, primarily active at the serotonin 2A site. Dopamine may contribute to LSD's effects more than is the case with other classical compounds, especially at later stages of the intoxication.

Scientists have synthesized interesting derivatives of LSD. MLD-41 and ALD-52 are psychedelic, whereas BOL-148 is not. This latter compound may be an effective treatment for cluster headaches—a disabling and difficult-to-treat pain syndrome.

DOSE AND ROUTE OF ADMINISTRATION

People take LSD nearly always orally, oftentimes ingesting small squares of LSD-saturated blotter paper. The minimal noticeable dose is 20–25 μg (micrograms). A fully psychedelic dose ranges from 100–500 μg, depending on one's sensitivity. Effects of oral LSD begin within fifteen to forty-five minutes, peak at three to six hours, and may last twelve or more hours. Tolerance to LSD occurs as with the other classical drugs. That is, after three or four days of daily dosing, subjective effects are minimal. After a comparable period of abstinence, normal sensitivity returns.

EFFECTS AND SIDE EFFECTS

As I discussed in Chapter 3, LSD is physically nontoxic and non-addictive. However, psychological toxicity may be significant in people who are inattentive to set and setting issues.

Because of the high morbidity of unsupervised use in the 1960s, LSD doses on the street gradually fell from 250–300 μg to 80 μg and lower, resulting in significantly fewer adverse effects. In addition, more sophisticated and safety-oriented approaches to taking LSD and other psychedelics have reduced the number and severity of adverse effects. I will address practical safety issues in detail in Chapter 11.

LEGAL

As much as any other drug, LSD was responsible for passage of the Controlled Substances Act of 1970. It resides in Schedule I, the most restrictive legal category, and comparable legislation around the world similarly prohibits it.

PSILOCYBIN

Psilocybin is having its moment in the sun. It is the psychedelic in greatest use within the research community and is at the forefront of decriminalization and legalization movements advocating for greater access to psychedelic substances. In addition, its presence in the natural world is leading to a greater awareness of both the "consciousness of nature" as well as of Indigenous cultures' use of these compounds.

HISTORY

Psilocybin occurs in "magic mushrooms," the consumption of which is cosmopolitan and extends deep into prehistory. Rock paintings in Spain and Algeria suggest that psilocybin species' use in the Old World may date as far back as 8000 BCE.

However, the Americas are where psychedelic mushrooms have made their greatest impression. Indigenous use in Latin America has occurred uninterruptedly for millennia in healing, shamanic, and spiritual settings. Archaeological evidence points to Mayan use of magic mushrooms between 500 BCE and 900 CE in Mexico and Central America. The Aztec word for psychedelic mushrooms is *teonanacatl*—"mushrooms of the gods" or "divine mushrooms." After the Spanish conquest of the Aztecs in the 1500s, ritual mushroom ceremonies continued underground among Mexican Mazatec and Zapotec peoples.

The Wassons—the banker R. Gordon and his pediatrician wife Valentina—rediscovered psychedelic mushroom ceremonies in the 1950s. A hugely popular *Life* magazine article described their experiences with an Indigenous Mexican healer, María Sabina.

Psilocybin thereafter saw use in psychiatry and psychopharmacology research, but it never attained the widespread popularity of LSD during the first wave of psychedelic enthusiasm. Researchers already had LSD and saw no advantage in shifting their attention away from it. In addition, the microscopic amounts of LSD necessary for a full experience facilitated the underground synthesis and distribution of enormous numbers of doses. Finally, there were no simple ways to grow psilocybin mushrooms, as there are today.

In the 1960s while at Harvard, Timothy Leary and his colleagues studied psilocybin. Leary's initial work with this compound helped establish the crucial concept of set and setting. In the Concord Prison Experiment, he administered psilocybin to prisoners in group psychotherapy, hoping to decrease prisoner recidivism after discharge. While initial results were encouraging, reanalysis of those data and longer-term follow-up demonstrated less impressive impact.

Also in the 1960s, Walter Pahnke, a psychiatrist at Harvard, administered psilocybin to divinity students in the Good Friday Experiment at Boston College's Marsh Chapel. He demonstrated that divinity students who received psilocybin were more likely to experience religious exaltation than those who received placebo.

We administered psilocybin in our University of New Mexico studies in the 1990s and reestablished its safety profile. Subsequent research at the University of Arizona demonstrated potential benefit in patients with obsessive-compulsive disorder. Several years later, Johns Hopkins researchers began their work giving psilocybin to normal volunteers in their clinical spirituality studies.

Because psilocybin occurs in the natural world, it has greater contemporary appeal than the synthetic LSD. It also is easy to grow psilocybin-containing mushrooms from spores that are available online and are legal in most jurisdictions. Several popular handbooks describe do-it-yourself procedures requiring minimal equipment and laboratory expertise.

Recently, the FDA has granted "breakthrough status" to psilocybin-assisted psychotherapy for treatment-resistant depression.[26] Other research studies suggest promise in treating patients with alcohol and tobacco addiction and end-of-life despair.

---

26. This designation expedites the development and review of a drug for treating a serious illness for which preliminary clinical evidence indicates the drug's superiority over current treatments.

BOTANY

Psilocybin-containing mushrooms occur throughout the world, numbering at least two hundred species. The most common genus is *Psilocybe*. Popular species are *P. cubensis*, *P. semilanceata*, *P. cyanescens*, and *P. azurescens*. The largest number of species are in Mexico, but they also grow wild—usually in humid subtropical forests—throughout the world.

While many psilocybin mushrooms species demonstrate a "bluing reaction" after bruising, this is not always the case. Typical concentrations of psilocybin in dried mushrooms are between 0.5–1 percent by weight. Mushroom caps contain more psilocybin than stems.

CHEMISTRY/PHARMACOLOGY

The chemical configuration of psilocybin is quite like that of DMT. It is 4-phosphoryloxy-DMT, a DMT molecule with a minor molecular addition. The body rapidly converts the non-psychoactive psilocybin to the psychoactive psilocin by removing the phosphate, resulting in 4-hydroxy-DMT. In other words, psilocybin is a "prodrug" for psilocin, being inactive itself. The pharmacology of psilocybin is like the other classical compounds—acting primarily on the serotonin 2A receptor—while the 5-HT1A subtype also appears to play a role.

Psilocybin provides the starting point for two synthetic psychedelic compounds: CEY-19 and CZ-74. The former is 4-phosphoryloxy-DET (diethyltryptamine) whereas the latter is 4-hydroxy-DET. The CEY compound is inactive and serves as a prodrug for the CZ one—like psilocybin serves as a prodrug for psilocin. Both are orally active and shorter acting than psilocybin/psilocin.

DOSE AND ROUTE OF ADMINISTRATION

The oral route is the most common way of consuming psilocybin. Low oral doses of pure psilocybin are 5 mg or less, and full doses are 25–30 mg. When consuming dried mushrooms, low doses are between 0.25–1 g, an average dose 1–2.5 g, and a high dose 2.5–5 g. However, sensitivity may vary. There are many recipes available for psilocybin tea. Other substances like cacao and honey may enhance absorption of psilocybin from mushrooms, but I am unaware of scientific data concerning this. We safely administered more than 50 mg to several subjects, whereas doses over 80 mg in two volunteers produced confusion and hyperthermia.

EFFECTS AND SIDE EFFECTS

Effects of oral psilocybin begin within fifteen to forty-five minutes, peak at one to two hours, plateau for about two hours, and are largely gone after six to eight hours. Other than the time course, the psilocybin experience is qualitatively like that of the other classical compounds LSD and mescaline. Tolerance to the psychological effects of psilocybin occurs after several days of daily dosing, and sensitivity returns after a comparable period of abstinence. Cross-tolerance occurs with LSD and mescaline, but not with DMT. That is, someone tolerant to LSD or mescaline will demonstrate a reduced response to psilocybin, and someone tolerant to psilocybin will demonstrate a reduced response to LSD or mescaline. However, someone psilocybin-tolerant will still respond fully to DMT.

LEGAL

Psilocybin and psilocin are Schedule I drugs. Mushrooms, as "carriers" of a prohibited substance, are also illegal, but not in every jurisdiction. For example, Amsterdam coffee shops and cafés serve psilocybin mushroom-containing food items, and psilocybin mushroom retreats are "not illegal" in Jamaica. Mushroom spores, since they do not contain psilocybin, are legal in most jurisdictions, but some states have prohibited them. I advise caution when considering partaking of psilocybin in "legal psilocybin mushroom churches" that claim protection under "religious freedom."

Psilocybin-containing mushrooms are at the forefront of movements to decriminalize and legalize psychedelics. Oregon has legalized "psilocybin products," and is establishing state-level regulatory and licensing boards for production, distribution, and administration. These legislative activities base themselves on preliminary data indicating efficacy of psilocybin-assisted psychotherapy in treatment-resistant depression and other conditions. However, the risk-benefit ratio of greater access remains uncertain.

DMT AND AYAHUASCA

Dimethyltryptamine, or DMT, is the simplest of the classical tryptamine psychedelics, not much larger than blood sugar or glucose. It is of great significance because of its presence in the mammalian brain. In addition, the Latin American DMT-containing brew, ayahuasca, is increasingly popular throughout the world. This interest has led to a surge in "ayahuasca tourism" in Latin America, legal ayahuasca-using churches in the West, underground "wellness" centers, and academic research into its psychotherapeutic potential.

HISTORY AND BOTANY

Indigenous Latin Americans have been using psychedelic snuffs and brews containing DMT for thousands of years.[27] Ayahuasca is a combination of two plants. The most common DMT-containing plant is *Psychotria viridis*. As DMT is orally inactive, it requires inhibition of the enzyme that breaks it down in the gut—monoamine oxidase or MAO. By a remarkable feat of pharmacology, Indigenous peoples in Latin America discovered the efficacy of combining the DMT-containing plant with one that inhibits MAO—*Banistereopsis caapi*. Syrian Rue—*Peganum harmala*—which grows

---

27. DMT is not the only psychedelic tryptamine in the snuffs and may even be absent. Two other tryptamines are also important: bufotenine and 5-methoxy-DMT.

in North America, also contains the MAO-inhibiting compounds necessary for oral DMT activity. Even pharmaceutical MAO-inhibiting drugs that see use for depression are effective in inhibiting DMT breakdown in the gut, resulting in "pharmahuasca." While DMT-containing and MAO-inhibiting plants usually form the basis of ayahuasca, sometimes the brew may not contain any DMT. Many other plants—for example, tobacco—play a role, depending on the intended effect.

Ayahuasca goes by several names depending on the setting of its use: for example, *caapi*, *daime*, *hoasca*, and *vegetal*. Ayahuasca is a Quechua word meaning "vine of the soul" or "vine of the dead." This points to its ability to provide access to normally invisible and immaterial worlds.

Anthropologists and botanists from the West first learned of ayahuasca's existence and properties in the mid-1800s, beginning with Richard Spruce. Richard Evans Schultes's field studies in the 1950s reignited interest in it, especially within the nascent psychedelic subculture.

Richard Manske in Canada first synthesized DMT in the 1930s as one of a series of novel tryptamines, but he did not study it. Latin American and US chemists eventually isolated DMT from psychedelic plants. Stephen Szára, a Hungarian psychiatrist and chemist, unable to obtain LSD from Sandoz from behind the Iron Curtain, discovered DMT's psychedelic properties in a series of self-experiments. Noticing no effect through increasingly large oral doses, he decided to inject it, and thus discovered its psychoactivity.

DMT remained a psychedelic niche drug for some time: short acting, intense, and active only after injection. Interest increased significantly, however, after its discovery in mammalian—including human—urine, spinal fluid, and blood.

The role of DMT in endogenous—that is, naturally occurring—psychoses was a major area of research during the first wave of human studies. Scientists sought to determine if DMT levels, formation, breakdown, or sensitivity differed between, say, schizophrenic patients and healthy subjects. Evidence supporting a role for endogenous DMT and naturally occurring psychoses was inconclusive by the time the CSA curtailed human psychedelic drug research. Despite calls for giving the DMT-psychosis theory a "decent burial" in the 1970s, this area remains of interest to scientists, especially in Europe.

The renewal of American clinical psychedelic drug research started with our five-year DMT project at the University of New Mexico that began in 1990.

CHEMISTRY/PHARMACOLOGY

In plants and animals, tryptophan is the first step in DMT synthesis. Plants produce their own tryptophan—an amino acid—but mammals must ingest it through the diet. One enzyme converts tryptophan into tryptamine, and another adds two methyl groups to tryptamine, resulting in di-methyl-tryptamine (dimethyltryptamine).

For years, scientists believed the lungs made DMT, but recent data indicate brain synthesis with minimal or no lung production. The theory of pineal synthesis of DMT, which I proposed in my 2001 book, remains inconclusive. A 2013 study reported its presence in living rodent pineal gland, but a 2019 study suggested that the previously reported pineal DMT instead came from the brain.

More important than whether the pineal makes DMT are the data demonstrating that the mammalian brain makes this psychedelic in concentrations similar to those of well-known neurotransmitters like serotonin and dopamine. This suggests the existence of a DMT neurotransmitter system. In addition, DMT levels increase in the dying rodent brain, especially in the visual cortex. This supports the idea that elevated levels of endogenous DMT contribute to the visual elements of the near-death state.

Laboratory synthesis of DMT is relatively simple, but the required chemicals are on the DEA "watch list." Therefore, the most common way of obtaining DMT for non-research purposes is by extracting it from DMT-rich plant material, frequently from *Mimosa hostilis* root bark.

The pharmacology of DMT is like other classical compounds. The serotonin 1A and sigma-1 receptors also play a role. A non-psychedelic analog of DMT—iso-DMT—is psychoplastogenic. DET (diethyltryptamine) and DPT (dipropyltryptamine) are two short-acting tryptamines that saw use during the first wave of human research. While both are active by injection, they have the added advantage of being orally active, with a duration of approximately two hours.

The primary MAO-inhibiting substances in ayahuasca belong to the beta-carboline family of compounds. These include harmine, harmaline, and tetrahydroharmine. These compounds by themselves possess psychoactive properties and likely contribute to the gastrointestinal side effects of the brew. However, their primary contribution is to allow DMT to become orally active. Taking oral DMT approximately twenty minutes after taking pure harmine or harmaline produces an orally active DMT experience.

Psychological tolerance to repeated frequent administration of DMT does not occur. We found no decrease in psychological effects after giving a full dose every thirty minutes four times in a morning. DMT does not exhibit cross-tolerance with other classical compounds, either. That is, an LSD- or psilocybin-tolerant person will still respond normally to a full dose of DMT.

A DETOUR THROUGH THE DMT ENDO-MATRIX

One of the most striking features of the full psychedelic experience is how real it feels—"more real than real." Does this mean that it is more real than real, or that it just feels that way? The presence of DMT in the mammalian brain and the possibility of a DMT neurotransmitter system point to a biological basis for our sense of reality.

I mentioned in Chapter 4—"How Psychedelics Work: The Brain"— that we discover the role of a neurotransmitter by observing changes brought about by drugs that modify that neurotransmitter's activity. In the case of serotonin, we have learned by the effects of SSRIs that this neurotransmitter is involved in impulse control and mood. Likewise, from the effects of dopamine-modifying drugs like amphetamine, we now know that dopamine regulates energy and reward. The hallmark of the DMT effect, on the other hand, is the feeling that what one is witnessing is more real than real, there is conviction of truth, meaning, what Dr. Freedman called "portentousness." Therefore, it is possible to imagine that DMT may regulate our sense of reality.

It is tempting to speculate that levels of DMT accompanying any experience—inner or outer—determine its meaningfulness for us. Is who we are—our sense of self, goals, truths, and values—simply a collection of DMT-reinforced events that come together in a more or less cohesive manner? If so, why do certain experiences increase DMT activity? We can suggest "stress," but this is circular reasoning. That is, if we define stress as that which increases DMT function, we still must understand why certain experiences are "stressful" and others are not.

Even more fanciful is the notion that we are all living in a DMT hallucination— one regulated by the maintenance of a normal range of DMT levels in the brain. This is not entirely far-fetched, either. I say this because there is no relationship between this world and the DMT world. The DMT experience completely replaces ongoing everyday experience. There is the DMT world and there is this one. The two appear to exist side by side. Whether you are interacting with one or the other depends on brain levels of DMT. One of our volunteers who received multiple DMT doses over several months described how it seemed that the DMT world was progressing along its own time course. Rather than entering the exact same "world" during study sessions, it felt as if he were visiting it after a week or two had elapsed there as well.

What then normally regulates DMT levels in our brains? And if "everyday" levels of endogenous DMT are responsible for maintaining everyday reality, how can we tell if we are simply living in a DMT simulation?

My answer—and I do not mean to be glib—is "Do nothing different." At this point, we have no way to know. Until we can turn off DMT synthesis and see what remains of our reality, this is all we have. In the meantime, cause and effect operate, we appear to have free will to decide this or that, so I suggest going about our lives in the same way as we always have.

DOSE AND ROUTE OF ADMINISTRATION

DMT is orally inactive and thus requires either smoking, snorting, or injecting. Smoking is the most common method, employing the freebase, which people vaporize and then inhale. DMT vape pens provide a less harsh smoking experience. When smoked or injected, effects begin within a couple of heartbeats, peak at two to ten minutes, and are barely noticeable at thirty to forty minutes. Ayahuasca effects begin at about thirty to sixty minutes, peak at two to three hours, and resolve over the next three to four hours. Vaporized DMT freebase is active at between 35–55 mg. People sometimes mistake DMT for 5-methoxy-DMT, which is ten times as potent; thus, one must make certain not to overdose on the latter compound believing it is the less potent DMT.

The amount of DMT in ayahuasca varies considerably depending on the specific brew. A low psychoactive dose of DMT in ayahuasca is about 30 mg, a medium dose 50 mg, and a high dose 70 mg and above. However, other studies have reported between 180–450 mg of DMT in a "dose." In addition, ayahuasca may be more or less concentrated, meaning a small volume of liquid may contain more DMT than a larger volume of more dilute material. Since estimates vary so widely, it makes sense to begin with a small amount of ayahuasca if you are not familiar with its effects.

EFFECTS AND SIDE EFFECTS

The first thing one notices after smoking or injecting DMT is a "rush," a sense of inner tension and acceleration. Rapidly with smoked DMT, and more gradually with an adequate dose of ayahuasca, one loses awareness of the body and responsiveness to the outside world. However, as opposed to the "K-hole" of high-dose ketamine intoxication (see page 133), if forced to move, one can. Once established, the DMT experience is highly visual with eyes open and especially when closed. Rapidly swirling, intensely saturated, and colored kaleidoscopic visual patterns may coalesce into more or less recognizable objects—for example, humanoid, insect-like, mechanical, or botanical "beings." DMT seems to produce "contact" with beings more often than the other classical psychedelics. These "entities" are aware of us, and mutual interactions take place. They may be benign or malevolent, and they often communicate with us verbally—usually telepathically from "mind to mind" rather than hearing an audible voice.

Smoked DMT produces robust increases in blood pressure and heart rate, and those with heart disease should avoid this route of administration. Ayahuasca also increases blood pressure and heart rate, but not as powerfully. In addition, nausea from the brew may lead to decreased heart rate and blood pressure. Another name for ayahuasca is "the purge," and vomiting and diarrhea are common even in those who use it regularly.

Studies of long-term ayahuasca users—mostly in the setting of ayahuasca religious organizations—provide reassuring data regarding long-term effects of regular use—three to five times per month for decades. General medical and psychiatric health and well-being are equal to or greater than those of matched controls. There is no evidence of brain damage; in fact, neuropsychological test scores are often better than those of matched controls. I have already mentioned a study that demonstrated increased thickness of certain parts of the cerebral cortex in long-term users, consistent with a psychoplastogenic effect.

Like psilocybin, ayahuasca produces rapid benefit in patients with depression and anxiety. DMT has begun seeing use as an antidepressant, and additional studies are determining its potential benefit in treatment of acute stroke and hastening functional recovery after a stroke.

LEGAL

Pure DMT is a Schedule I drug. However, the use of ayahuasca in the US by two Brazil-based churches is legal. The US Supreme Court ruled unanimously in 2006 to protect the religious use of ayahuasca for one of these churches, the UDV.[28] Several years later, federal courts similarly granted an exemption for ayahuasca use in another church, the Santo Daime.[29]

"THE TOAD"—5-METHOXY-DMT (5-MEO-DMT)

The compound 5-methoxy-DMT occurs in many Latin American psychoactive plants, especially those that see use in psychedelic snuffs. Two such are *Anadenanthera colubrina* and *A. peregrina*. *Cebil* and *vilca* are Indigenous names for snuffs that come from the former plant, and *yopo* and *parica* for those which come from the latter. In addition, the Sonoran Desert, or Colorado River, toad produces a venom in its parotid glands rich in 5-MeO-DMT. Until recently, the name for this toad was *Bufo alvarius*, but changes in classification now identify it as *Incilius alvarius*. As old habits die hard, I will continue referring to the toad as "Bufo." Both psychedelic snuffs and toad venom are also rich in bufotenine (alternative spelling: bufotenin).

---

28. In Portuguese: União do Vegetal—"The union of the plants."
29. "Holy Daime." In Portuguese, *daime* means "give me."

HISTORY

While archaeological evidence suggests the use of toad venom in Mesoamerican culture dating back more than three thousand years, this is less certain than the importance of psychedelic snuffs in these cultures. Traditional Latin American healers continue to use toad venom, but the extent of Indigenous use is unknown.

For years, 5-MeO-DMT was an obscure compound. However, increasing use and the threats such use pose to the toad have significantly raised its profile. Laboratory synthesis of 5-MeO-DMT is not difficult and offers a reliable alternative to "toad-milking." This is like the overharvesting of mescaline-containing peyote, with a comparable movement to use synthetic mescaline.

Japanese chemists synthesized 5-MeO-DMT in the 1930s, and papers from the 1950s described its presence in Bufo skin. However, it was not until 1983 that the modern era of 5-MeO-DMT and the toad began when Albert Most published his booklet *Bufo alvarius: The Psychedelic Toad of the Sonoran Desert*. Nine years later, following up on Most's findings, Wade Davis and Andrew Weil published a paper describing the effects of self-administration of the smoked venom.

Bufotenine occurs in both toad venom and psychedelic snuffs. Clinical research with this compound occurred in the 1950s. After intravenous injection, its psychedelic effects were equivocal, while cardiovascular side effects were significant. More recent data suggest fewer psychedelic effects using the smoked or snorted routes of administration than those occurring with injection.

CHEMISTRY/PHARMACOLOGY

Unlike other classical tryptamine psychedelics, 5-MeO-DMT is more active at the serotonin 1A site than the 2A. Both bufotenine and 5-MeO-DMT appear to be endogenous to humans and other mammals. However, the details and specific location of their synthesis are not as well understood as is the case with DMT. 5-MeO-DMT, like other tryptamine psychedelics, is psychoplastogenic.

Parotid gland secretions of Bufo may contain 5–15 percent of 5-MeO-DMT by dry weight in addition to other compounds of varying psychoactivity and toxicity. Assuming 10 percent 5-MeO-DMT by dry weight, 100 mg of venom would provide a 10 mg dose of 5-MeO-DMT.

We know less about tolerance to repeated, closely spaced administration of 5-MeO-DMT than with DMT. In animals, tolerance to some drug effects occur, whereas tolerance to other effects does not. A report in cats suggested sensitization—that is, greater responses to the same dose with repeated dosing.

DOSE AND ROUTES OF ADMINISTRATION

People administer the toad venom by the smoked route, and pure 5-MeO-DMT by smoking the free base or snorting a water-soluble salt. The snorted pure drug is active at 3–5 mg, a full dose being between 10–20 mg. Vaporized and inhaled 5-MeO-DMT is active at 1–2 mg, an average dose is 5–10 mg, and a high dose is 10–20 mg. Note that these doses are approximately five to ten times less than those for DMT, and one must be careful to distinguish between the two so as not to overdose on the more potent compound. It is not uncommon for people to think that what they are smoking is DMT when it is actually 5-MeO-DMT.

The time course of pure 5-MeO-DMT is like that of DMT. The smoked drug begins working within a few heartbeats, peaks at two to six minutes, and resolves by thirty to forty-five minutes. 5-MeO-DMT vape pens provide an easier-to-control dosing regimen, like DMT-containing ones. Snorted 5-MeO-DMT comes on within a couple of minutes, peaks at ten to twenty minutes, and resolves within an hour.

The one clinical laboratory research study of 5-MeO-DMT I am aware of used the vaporized and inhaled compound, and there were no effects on blood pressure or heart rate. This is surprising, as I would expect that in most cases, the psychological reaction alone would elevate these parameters. Without additional research data, it seems prudent to avoid using 5-MeO-DMT if one suffers from heart disease.

There are no controlled clinical studies using 5-MeO-DMT for psychiatric disorders.

EFFECTS/SIDE EFFECTS

The subjective effects of 5-MeO-DMT usually differ from those of DMT. The DMT state is full of content—especially visions—and the maintenance of one's personality with which one interacts with that content. In addition, time and space continue, albeit in a highly modified manner. On the other hand, the 5-MeO-DMT experience is typically "ego-dissolving," "white light," and absent normal experiences of time and space. This experience of breaking down one's sense of self and merging with all existence, while desirable for some, can be traumatic in others, especially with an inadvertent overdose and poor preparation. Complete amnesia for the experience is not rare, during which one might scream, thrash, sing, or dance. Therefore, it is particularly important to have a sober "sitter" when using this substance.

The "annihilation of the ego" may be responsible for the more frequent occurrence of flashbacks after 5-MeO-DMT use. One study reported that almost 70 percent of 5-MeO-DMT smokers reported these "reactivations," or flashbacks. Some consider such symptoms—unbidden reoccurrences of certain elements of a previous psychedelic experience—pleasurable. For others, however, they are quite unpleasant, manifesting as intense panic attacks, sometimes in the middle of the night. They may be slow to resolve and difficult to treat. While some suggest "getting back on the horse" right away—that is, smoking the substance again—I do not recommend this.

LEGAL

The pure drug 5-MeO-DMT is a Schedule I substance in the US State laws vary regarding possession of Bufo and/or its secretions, but nearly all consider it illegal to collect the toad and/or its venom with the intent to use the venom as a psychedelic. In addition, transporting the toad across state lines is illegal. Several states have labeled the toad as endangered or threatened because of the increased popularity of the venom.

IBOGAINE

Ibogaine is a tryptamine psychedelic with a more complex chemical structure and pharmacology than the classical tryptamines like psilocybin and DMT. It also possesses unique anti-addiction properties. Ibogaine is the primary psychoactive alkaloid in several species of *Tabernanthe* shrubs and trees in Central Africa. The most well known of these is *Tabernanthe iboga*.

HISTORY

The Pygmies may have first discovered the psychoactive effects of iboga. The Bwiti religion of Gabon currently uses the plant in their religious ceremonies. The first initiatory experience sometimes lasts for days, involves massive doses of root bark, and may rarely result in death. If the initiation is successful, one "breaks open the head." After completing the Bwiti initiation, acolytes take smaller doses in regular ceremonies.

Botanists first described iboga in the late 1890s. Chemists isolated ibogaine in the early 1900s, but synthesis of ibogaine did not occur until the 1960s. The French—who had colonized Gabon—marketed an iboga extract that saw use as a stimulant from the early- to the mid-1900s. Dosages ranged from 8–30 mg.

In the 1960s, heroin addict Howard Lotsof took ibogaine for its psychedelic effects, and he serendipitously discovered its ability to markedly reduce—and sometimes entirely abolish—withdrawal symptoms and subsequent craving. An extensive underground network of ibogaine therapists began using it to treat addictions: cocaine, amphetamine and methamphetamine, alcohol, opiates, and tobacco. Low-dose studies of ibogaine began at the University of Miami in the early 1990s. However, the FDA ended this research after concerns grew over the drug's cardiovascular and neurological toxicity. Nevertheless, ibogaine clinics currently exist in several countries and advertise widely online.

Thousands of patients have received ibogaine for the treatment of opioid- or other substance-use disorders, but there are yet no adequate well-controlled clinical trials. These less-than-gold standard studies are uniformly positive, however, suggesting rapid resolution of withdrawal symptoms, reduced craving, and extended abstinence.

CHEMISTRY/PHARMACOLOGY

Ibogaine and noribogaine—its primary psychoactive metabolite—are pharmacologically complex. They interact with other receptors in addition to the serotonin 2A and 1A types. The kappa opioid site is important in ibogaine's mechanism of action, and it is of interest that salvinorin A, which I discuss in Chapter 10, also interacts robustly with this site. Ibogaine and noribogaine also modify the activity of mu opioid receptors (to which traditional opiates like morphine bind), serotonin reuptake mechanisms, and the NMDA receptor. This latter site is the primary one upon which ketamine acts.

Ibogaine in laboratory animals reduces opiate self-administration as well as withdrawal symptoms. It also blocks self-administration of alcohol, cocaine, and nicotine. The psychoplastogenic effects of ibogaine involve brain growth factors, as do those of the classical compounds. A non-psychedelic analog of ibogaine, TBG, is also psychoplastogenic and demonstrates efficacy in animal models of depression, anxiety, and addiction.

The length of time ibogaine remains in the blood is significantly shorter than that of noribogaine—two to six hours compared to twenty-four to thirty hours. As the cardiovascular effects of ibogaine occur at the late stages of intoxication, it is likely that the metabolite is more toxic to the heart than the parent compound.

Early reports of ibogaine neurotoxicity in monkeys, in particular in the cerebellum—a brain area near the back of the head responsible for coordinated movement—raised alarms among federal regulators.[30] These data, along with reports of ibogaine-related deaths in uncontrolled settings, led the FDA to end early clinical studies with the drug. Subsequent research demonstrated a lack of neurotoxicity, and it is likely that very high doses of the drug, and/or species differences, contributed to those original data.

DOSE AND ROUTE OF ADMINISTRATION

People take ibogaine orally. Published reports of human ibogaine studies suffer from uncertainty regarding the dose of drug because of large variations in concentrations of ibogaine in iboga root bark. For example, one sees papers describing concentrations of 0.6–11 percent, 7 percent, 8–30 percent, and 74 percent. Therefore, it is much easier to calculate the dose using pure synthetic ibogaine.

In the clinic, opiate- and/or cocaine-dependent patients receive between 5–30 mg/kg of pure ibogaine. A high dose is in the range of 12 mg/kg and above. In some settings, patients receive smaller, gradually increasing, doses of ibogaine spread out over several days. This reportedly produces fewer side effects.

---

30. Interestingly, the cerebellum also regulates repetitive behaviors, which may be relevant to its anti-addiction effects.

EFFECTS/SIDE EFFECTS

Onset is relatively slow, between one to three hours, and effects may last for twenty-four hours. There is a typical psychedelic state that predominates for approximately the first six hours, corresponding to high concentrations of ibogaine in the blood. Ibogaine levels drop off rapidly and noribogaine levels then rise. Noribogaine remains in the blood for at least another twelve to twenty-four hours. The effects of this latter compound most likely mediate the decreased withdrawal and craving that follow the early psychedelic part of the experience. The resolution of all effects is slow, and there is a prolonged afterglow often lasting for weeks.

Ibogaine causes ataxia—unsteadiness while walking. This may reflect its cerebellar effects. It is advisable to remain seated or lying down for the duration of the experience. When getting up to use the bathroom, for example, make certain to have someone help you. Nausea and vomiting may occur more often than with other classical compounds.

The cardiovascular effects of ibogaine—probably related to noribogaine—are due to its prolonging the "QT interval," an electrical process regulating cardiac rhythm. An abnormal QT interval may result in a dangerously low heart rate, arrhythmias, and death. It is likely that low levels of potassium and magnesium contribute to the cardiac toxicity of ibogaine, which points to the necessity of careful medical screening and monitoring when using ibogaine in detoxification protocols. Thus, it is not surprising that all ibogaine-related deaths have occurred in nonmedical settings.

DEATHS

We know of about three dozen ibogaine-related deaths. The largest study to date of two hundred patients under careful medical supervision reported no serious adverse effects nor fatalities. In cases of fatalities, a range of complicating factors were most likely involved: questionable purity of the drug; very large doses; poor health of patients; and the presence of drugs that could interfere with ibogaine metabolism or, on their own, produce heart rhythm abnormalities. In addition, the metabolism of ibogaine is variable within the general population, and some individuals may metabolize it much more slowly than others, leading to dangerous increases in concentration of the parent compound and/or metabolite.

LEGAL

Ibogaine, but not the iboga plant, is classified as Schedule I in the US and several other countries. Ibogaine clinics operate within a legal "gray area" in, for example, Mexico, Canada, and Europe. Export of the plant from Gabon is illegal.

CHAPTER 8

MDMA

MDMA stands for 3,4-methylenedioxymethamphetamine. The term "empathogen" or "entactogen" indicates its unique constellation of psychological effects. These differ from the classical compounds in that perceptual alterations and disruption of the normal sense of self are significantly less pronounced with MDMA than are its emotional properties.

MDMA is a phenethylamine, a family of compounds to which both the psychedelic mescaline and non-psychedelic amphetamines belong. Its popular name is "ecstasy." "Molly" also refers to MDMA but is a term that may also apply to substances containing additional non-MDMA compounds or no MDMA at all.[31]

The German pharmaceutical company Merck synthesized MDMA in the 1910s as an agent to stop abnormal bleeding, but it never saw clinical use. It languished until Alexander Shulgin synthesized it again in the 1970s and described its psychological effects. Shulgin shared it with the psychedelic psychologist Leo Zeff. Soon thereafter, Leo began employing it as an adjunct to individual and group psychotherapy and trained many therapists in its use. Later in the 1970s, MDMA became a popular party drug in urban centers and as an aid to psychotherapy in the psychedelic underground.

MDMA's increased use and neurotoxic effects prompted the DEA to emergency schedule it in the mid-1980s. Attempts to reverse this decision

---

31. For example, ketamine, "bath salts," amphetamines, caffeine, opiates, ephedrine, and LSD.

by a network of scientists, scholars, and MDMA-using therapists drew major media attention. This resulted in a massive increase in the drug's popularity with no effect on its permanent placement into Schedule I.

The FDA has granted breakthrough status for MDMA in the treatment of post-traumatic stress disorder. In addition, preliminary reports suggest efficacy in social anxiety in adults with autism spectrum, as well as in alcoholism.

PSYCHOPHARMACOLOGY

Acute effects of MDMA result from the release of dopamine, serotonin, and norepinephrine from presynaptic nerve cells, and reduced reuptake of these neurotransmitters. MDMA-induced elevations of the prosocial hormone oxytocin may also contribute to its unique psychological properties. Effects on the amygdala, a brain center involved in fear, may mediate MDMA's ability to help one deal with negative emotions. For example, the amygdala reacts less robustly to threatening images and more robustly to positive ones under MDMA's influence. This may explain how MDMA allows for the recovery and processing of fearful memories with less fear. In addition, MDMA reduces threat perception and/or increases the relevance of reward and social interactions.

DOSE AND ROUTES OF ADMINISTRATION

Most people take MDMA orally. Recreational users may snort it, which leads to a faster onset, more intense peak, and shorter duration. Typical oral doses range between 80–150 mg. Frequently, people take a "booster," usually one-half of the original dose, 90–150 minutes after the initial dose. This prolongs the altered state and provides a more gradual resolution of effects. Responses to oral administration begin in about thirty to forty minutes, peak at ninety minutes to three hours, and are mostly over by five to six hours, but may extend up to eight hours if one uses a booster. It is important to not continue boosting in either therapy or nonmedical settings, because this is where side effects began to predominate over pleasurable ones.

EFFECTS/SIDE EFFECTS

MDMA's properties are primarily emotional and physical. One may feel more open, euphoric, sexually and/or mentally aroused, accepting, unafraid, relaxed, and clearheaded. There is a magnification of sensations and a desire to intensify them by dancing, talking, or touching. People experience increased sociability and closeness with others, plus greater self-confidence, interpersonal warmth, and empathy.

Visual effects are modest. There may be brightening of lights and a sparkling in the air. Part of this is due to MDMA enlarging pupil diameter. Some people use smaller doses as aids to study, create, or meditate, like the use of amphetamines or methylphenidate.

As with other psychedelics, effects are dependent on set and setting. While individual or small group settings may promote relaxation and enhanced communication, large dance venues may lead to increased activity and a self-absorbed state.

Users may take other drugs with MDMA; for example, combining MDMA with LSD—"candy-flipping"—reduces the anxiety that may come from LSD without reducing its other effects. Other drugs include ketamine, mushrooms, and 2C-B—a phenethylamine with more psychedelic properties than MDMA but less than those of mescaline. Common acute side effects of typical doses include double and blurred vision from dilated pupils and/or nystagmus—uncontrolled rapid back-and-forth eye movements. In addition, one may experience restlessness, teeth grinding, elevated temperature, muscle cramps, chills, rapid heart rate, increased blood pressure, nausea/vomiting, insomnia, erectile dysfunction, and sweating. Death may occur from hyperthermia due to overheating and dehydration, especially in a hot, crowded club setting. Drinking only water without replacing electrolytes may cause decreased sodium levels, which may lead to seizures.

For the next few days after taking MDMA, some describe feeling sad, irritable, impulsive, angry, unable to experience pleasure, depressed, or anxious. They may experience poor concentration and have difficulty sleeping, difficulty thinking, decreased appetite, and diminished sex drive and/or function.

TOLERANCE AND ADDICTION

I am unaware of clinical research studies investigating tolerance to MDMA in humans. Thus, we are dependent on data that researchers collect "in the field," where they have little control over crucial factors like the purity and doses of MDMA people take. Nevertheless, those uncontrolled data point to tolerance to MDMA's psychological effects with regular heavy use. This means that to achieve the same pleasurable psychological effects, one must take higher doses over time. While psychological effects diminish with regular use, cardiovascular and temperature effects do not, and this raises the risk of medical problems emerging with ever-increasing doses. In addition, anecdotal reports frequently note that one never feels the same effects after the first MDMA experience, even with limited infrequent use.

It is unclear whether MDMA "addiction" occurs with a distinct physical withdrawal syndrome like that of opiates and alcohol. However, psychological withdrawal occurs in recreational users, and the greater the use, the more symptoms. These include drug craving, fatigue, decreased appetite and mood, sexual dysfunction, depression, and poor concentration.

A unique potential adverse effect of MDMA is the "serotonin syndrome." This results from a toxic level of MDMA-stimulated serotonin in the synapse. Mild symptoms are restlessness, tremor, shivering, diarrhea, increased blood pressure and heart rate, and unsteadiness. In severe cases one sees elevated body temperature, muscle rigidity, confusion, seizures, and coma. Some cases are fatal.

No cases of serotonin syndrome have occurred in any clinical trials. Rather, it may occur when people take MDMA in combination with other serotonin-active drugs. These include amphetamines, opioids (especially tramadol), cocaine, both SSRI and SNRI[32] antidepressants, antihistamines, atypical antipsychotics, prescription MAO inhibitors, and the antibiotic linezolid.

NEUROTOXICITY

Neurotoxic, or brain damaging, effects of MDMA have dogged its use since the mid-1980s. Many advocates for MDMA use, especially as an adjunctive treatment for psychotherapy, minimize these effects. They refer to patients taking "nontoxic" doses; inconsistent results from brain-imaging studies; impure, adulterated, or counterfeit MDMA; even if these abnormalities exist, they normalize with prolonged abstinence; differences between humans' and nonhuman species' sensitivity to the drug; and uncontrolled settings for its use. Nevertheless, neurotoxicity of MDMA is not a trivial issue, and it is an important consideration when deciding whether to take MDMA, in what setting, how much, and how often.

---

32. Serotonin-norepinephrine reuptake inhibitors. The most well known are duloxetine and venlafaxine.

When making this decision, keep in mind the notion of the risk-benefit ratio. What are the potential benefits relative to the potential risks? In cases of severe PTSD for which no other treatments have helped, and for which evidence points to two or three MDMA plus psychotherapy sessions providing significant benefit, this ratio is favorable. On the other hand, recreational heavy use every weekend in combination with alcohol and other drugs in an overheated environment—a bar, house party, or nightclub—carries more risk than benefit. In between lies regular but infrequent use—say, monthly or several times a year—for creative, psychotherapeutic, partner intimacy, or spiritual purposes.

The long-term neurotoxicity is related to the same mechanisms responsible for acute psychological effects. That is, after too much or too frequent MDMA-induced neurotransmitter release and reuptake blockade, the relevant nerve endings die back. A frequent finding is long-term impairment of serotonin synthesis and reuptake, which may reflect damage to serotonin-containing neurons. Data for dopamine and norepinephrine are less consistent. The conversion of orally administered MDMA to MDA—3,4-methylenedioxyamphetamine—may be primarily responsible for these neurotoxic effects. If one injects MDMA directly into the brain— which bypasses MDA production—there is less neurotoxicity.[33] Both the neurological/brain imaging and clinical deficits may improve with long-term abstinence.

Since we have been discussing neurotoxicity, let me address the issue of MDMA "draining spinal fluid" from users. MDMA does not reduce the amount of spinal fluid in the nervous system. Rather, it was scientists performing spinal taps on research subjects—to measure levels of various neurotransmitters—that "drained" spinal fluid. And the amount of fluid involved was minuscule.

---

33. Development of MDMA-like compounds that do not convert to MDA may possess a greater safety profile than MDMA.

LEGAL

MDMA is a Schedule I drug.

SUMMARY

I treat the adverse effects of no other drug in this handbook in as much detail as I do with MDMA. The dividing line between the "right amount" of MDMA and "too much" is indistinct. My conclusions about MDMA are as follows: For those interested in psychedelic drugs, but afraid of having too intense, disorienting, or destabilizing an experience with classical compounds, MDMA may serve as a milder entry into these altered states. In addition, MDMA may have unique therapeutic properties. However, I wonder if small doses of classical compounds might be just as effective. For example, in our DMT work, we found that the amount of vasopressin in the blood rose to extremely high levels after drug administration. Vasopressin is closely related to oxytocin, the prosocial hormone that may mediate the empathy and emotional closeness resulting from MDMA. Unfortunately, researchers have not systematically compared the psychological effects of MDMA and low doses of non-neurotoxic classical compounds. If low doses of classical drugs were similarly effective, their use would raise no concern about neurotoxicity.

It is probably safe to take pure MDMA in small to moderate doses a handful of times in one's life, perhaps even just once. However, regular, frequent, and heavy use is only asking for trouble.

CHAPTER 9

KETAMINE

Ketamine is the first legally approved psychedelic for clinical use; specifically, as an add-on pharmacotherapy for treatment-resistant depression. However, it is not a classical psychedelic like LSD or psilocybin. Its subjective effects are similar to those of the classical compounds, but its pharmacology differs, and its psychological and physical risks are greater than those of the classical drugs.

Other names for ketamine include "K," "Special K," and the trade name Ketalar. Ketamine is a synthetic drug and belongs to the class of arylcyclohexylamines. Researchers developed ketamine in the 1960s as an alternative to PCP. PCP, or phencyclidine ("angel dust"), was an effective anesthetic but quickly became a drug of abuse. Chemists at Parke-Davis (now part of Pfizer) persevered and after making minor molecular modifications, discovered ketamine.

I saw numerous cases of PCP intoxication when I worked in the Sacramento County hospital emergency room in the 1970s. People under its influence were confused, paranoid, and because of its pain-blocking effects, possessed superhuman strength. We knew someone was on PCP when it took at least four burly police officers—one for each limb—to pin a patient to the gurney and tie them down. Convulsions and cardiac toxicity sometimes led to coma and death. Ketamine was much safer than PCP and first saw use in combat situations during the Vietnam War.

Ketamine is useful in anesthesia because it does not lower blood pressure nor decrease the drive to breathe. Ketamine remains a popular anesthetic agent because of its intense pain-suppressing, as well as immobilizing, effects. These are valuable properties for working with children or in burn units. These characteristics also make it a popular veterinary anesthetic. It is effective for acute and chronic pain management as well, like opiates, but less prone to abuse.

At sub-anesthetic doses, ketamine causes "emergence phenomena," which resemble the subjective effects of classical psychedelics. Its use in psychiatry began in 2000, when Yale researchers discovered the rapid antidepressant effects of psychedelic doses of ketamine. Research continues into its antidepressant properties.

PHARMACOLOGY

Ketamine and its most important metabolite HNK (hydroxynorketamine) exert their effects by blocking N-methyl-D-aspartate (NMDA) receptors. These receptors are a primary target of the neurotransmitter glutamate. This differs from the classical psychedelics, where serotonin plays the dominant role. Ketamine and HNK also stimulate neuroplasticity and neurogenesis. In addition, the mTOR—"mechanistic target of rapamycin"[34]—pathway is important in ketamine's antidepressant action, as is the sigma-1 receptor.

Data regarding the functional connectivity effects of ketamine are inconsistent but generally are like those we see with the classical drugs. These include increased brain entropy, increased global connectivity, decreased top-down and increased bottom-up activity.

---

34. The mTOR enzyme regulates a host of cellular processes and structures, including insulin effects.

Ketamine's psychoplastogenic effects begin quickly in animal models, within sixty to ninety minutes after exposure. However, these effects, while continuing for over two weeks, do not last as long as those of classical psychedelics.

The overlap between symptoms of schizophrenia and the sub-anesthetic ketamine "psychedelic" state has led to studies similar to those that investigated the relationship between classical psychedelics and psychosis. In normal volunteers, ketamine produces "negative" symptoms of schizophrenia; e.g., lethargy, reduced emotional capacity, and reduced speech. Classical psychedelics, on the other hand, produce "positive" symptoms like paranoia, delusions, and hallucinations. Administering ketamine to schizophrenic patients worsens both positive and negative symptoms. This type of research may lead to novel treatments for psychosis, ones that target the receptor mechanisms mediating the ketamine-induced altered state. This is similar to how the relationship between LSD and psychosis helped us develop new antipsychotic medications. That is, drugs that block the LSD effect have antipsychotic efficacy in psychosis. Likewise, developing drugs that block ketamine's "psychotomimetic" effects may turn out to be clinically useful.

DOSE AND ROUTES OF ADMINISTRATION

Ketamine is active by multiple routes. Oral, sublingual, intramuscular, nasal, and intravenous are the most common medical ones. Snorting and intramuscular injection are the most popular nonmedical recreational routes.

Effects of nasal ketamine—either recreationally snorting dried powder or nasal sprays for medical use—begin within three to five minutes and last about thirty to sixty minutes. Recreational "bumps" of ketamine powder range between 30–100 mg, and doses of Spravato[35] for antidepressant treatment are either 56 or 84 mg.

Intramuscular ketamine doses for depression range from 0.5–2 mg/kg. Effects begin within three to five minutes and last about an hour. Intravenous ketamine for depression delivers the drug as an infusion over forty minutes and uses similar doses. Effects begin within thirty seconds and cease about ten minutes after the infusion ends. Doses of oral ketamine that produce a moderately intense psychedelic effect range from 100–300 mg. "Psycholytic" doses of ketamine for individual or couples psychotherapy range from 50–150 mg sublingual or oral. Lozenges appear superior to swallowed preparations. Effects begin at about five minutes and last about one to two hours. Rectal administration of a ketamine suppository is occasionally necessary to reduce nausea and vomiting and/or if patients have difficulty swallowing. For depression treatment, patients usually wear eyeshades and listen to clinician-selected music.

We mostly hear about treatment models using doses and routes of administration that produce at least a moderately altered state. However, some clinicians use minimally or non-psychoactive oral or sublingual doses of ketamine for depression and/or pain. Treatment may be daily or simply as needed.

In psychotherapeutic settings, clinicians may administer a booster—oral, sublingual, or intramuscular—of half the original dose as effects begin to subside. This is like MDMA boosting, either in a psychotherapeutic or recreational context.

---

35. Spravato is an *isomer* of ketamine and requires special registration to prescribe and administer. An isomer is either the "right-hand" or "left-hand" version of a molecule, like one's right and left hands. Sometimes one isomer is more effective than the other or possesses fewer side effects. At other times, drug companies simply market one isomer for patent purposes. Spravato is the S- ("left-hand") isomer: "esketamine."

SUBJECTIVE EFFECTS

Low doses of ketamine feel like alcohol or sedatives—slurred speech, relaxation and reduction of anxiety, pleasure and euphoria, a dreamy feeling, giddiness, incoordination, and lack of balance. The pleasurable effects of low-dose ketamine—which some compare to MDMA—contribute to its popularity as a club drug. One may also use low doses to function in everyday situations—shopping, normal socializing, and school—like a benzodiazepine antianxiety agent. Creativity and problem-solving may improve.

At psychedelic doses, one experiences changes in the consistency of the body—as if it consists of wood or plastic—distorted body parts or shape, and a feeling of weightlessness, floating, or hovering. Visions, ecstatic emotions, new insights, and auditory distortions are common at psychedelic doses.

High doses of ketamine may cause one to enter the "K-hole." Imagine being under general anesthesia—unable to move or open the eyes—but still being conscious. It is a state of mute immobility, dissociation, and sensory detachment. It may feel as if one is melting into his/her surroundings, disconnected from reality, with no sense of self. The world appears deep within one's consciousness, full of visual and auditory contents. One may enter the white light. Balls of energy and color represent people or "beings," and one may find oneself in deep outer space. Some people find the K-hole extraordinarily appealing, while for others who are not prepared, it is a terrifying ordeal.

Studies suggest that the K-hole is like the naturally occurring near-death experience. There is an initial buzzing or ringing sound, travel through a dark tunnel at high speed toward a bright light, the conviction of being dead, and telepathy with spiritual beings.

THERAPEUTIC USES

Dozens of research studies have demonstrated that ketamine improves mood rapidly in patients with depression who have not responded well to traditional antidepressant or other therapies. This is similar to what we see with classical psychedelic treatments such as psilocybin and ayahuasca. Nevertheless, it is not a miracle cure, and reports of increased depression, suicidal ideation, and questionable efficacy counter such claims. In addition, there is a substantial literature supporting ketamine treatment for acute and/or chronic pain, even in those who either no longer respond to opiates or have developed an opiate dependency problem. Preliminary data indicate potential benefit in those with alcohol dependence and bulimia. While improving depression in patients with PTSD, it may not be effective for the core PTSD symptoms. Ketamine quickly reduces suicidal impulses and is seeing use in emergency room settings for that purpose. Some law enforcement agencies employ ketamine to "chemically restrain" unruly detainees.

How much, and what type, of psychotherapy to administer alongside ketamine administration for depression and other psychiatric disorders is an open question. In fact, one of the attractive elements of modern "ketamine therapy" is how biological effects may take precedence over psychological ones. This contrasts with the debate concerning the classical compounds, where the model is "psychedelic-assisted psychotherapy" rather than simply a "biological" treatment. Nevertheless, there is evidence in both research and nonacademic settings that psychotherapy in combination with ketamine is more effective than ketamine alone and produces fewer adverse effects.

The Spravato—proprietary nasal administration of ketamine—program involves twice-weekly dosing for a month, then weekly for the next month, with long-term treatment being every one to two weeks thereafter. The typical spacing of treatments for ketamine outside of the Spravato program ranges from one to five weeks.

Ketamine clinics are an increasingly common site in metropolitan areas, run by nurse practitioners, anesthesiologists, psychiatrists, or family practitioners. Some clinics include psychotherapy and others do not. During the COVID pandemic, clinics have been selling mail-order ketamine lozenges, and if therapy is involved, may do so remotely.

Spravato is expensive, but more insurance companies are reimbursing treatment. Generic ketamine is inexpensive, and compounding pharmacies can prepare ketamine spray for significantly less cost than out-of-pocket expenses for Spravato. In addition, one does not need to be a registered Spravato provider to prescribe generic ketamine through a compounding pharmacy.

ADVERSE EFFECTS

Ketamine possesses an array of acute and long-term adverse effects that do not occur with the classical compounds. It is more prone to both abuse and physical side effects.

PHYSICAL

Higher doses of ketamine raise blood pressure and heart rate and may worsen cardiac symptoms in the presence of heart disease. Ketamine also increases intraocular pressure and may cause problems in people with glaucoma. Other unwanted effects are not uncommon, especially with recreational use. These include dizziness, salivation, nausea, vomiting, and double vision resulting from nystagmus. Decreased body sensation may be dangerous if one needs to be aware of pain. Deaths due directly to ketamine alone are rare. However, deaths due to accidents may occur; for example, lying in a bathtub unable to lift one's head out of the water. A friend died in those circumstances. In addition, if one vomits and cannot turn their head to the side, they may inhale their vomit and aspirate.

Longer-term adverse effects of recreational use include urinary problems, especially inflammation of the bladder, as well as gastrointestinal cramping. The urinary bladder effects may also occur with Spravato. Neurotoxicity occurs at higher doses, neuroprotection and other beneficial effects at lower doses. It appears as if ketamine is more neurotoxic to the developing brain than to the adult one.

PSYCHOLOGICAL

Amnesia and forgetfulness may occur with long-term heavy recreational use, as may paranoia and mood swings. Adverse psychological effects of mind-altering doses of ketamine in a medical setting are uncommon but may include increased suicidal ideation and worsening depression. Note that these adverse effects may also occur with traditional antidepressants as well as with psilocybin treatment.

Recreational ketamine addiction occurs not infrequently. Tolerance to the psychological effects may require doses six to seven times greater than those with which someone has begun, and frequent users may take the drug until they run out. Famous cases of out-of-control ketamine use include the psychiatrist John Lilly—famous for his work with dolphin-human communication and isolation tanks—and Marcia Moore—author of *Journeys into the Bright World*. Physical withdrawal is less well established than psychological withdrawal.

Ketamine may be mixed with or entirely substitute for cocaine or MDMA. Mixtures of ketamine and other drugs can be particularly dangerous. For example, combining a stimulant/cocaine with ketamine will lead to increased activity but in the setting of poor motor control, and combining it with alcohol would amplify the sedating and other disinhibiting effects. Ketamine's immobilizing effects sometimes see use as a date-rape drug.

LEGAL

Ketamine is a Schedule III drug and requires only a normal prescribing license. However, it is illegal to possess ketamine for nonmedical use, or to sell or distribute it.

CHAPTER 10

SALVIA DIVINORUM/ SALVINORIN A

Salvinorin A is the primary psychoactive compound in *Salvia divinorum*. This unassuming plant goes by various names, including "diviners' mint," "diviners' sage," "ska pastora" (sage/mint of the shepherdess), "yerba de la pastora" (herb of the shepherdess), and "Maria pastora" (Mary the shepherdess). It is an odorless member of the mint family and grows in the mountains of Oaxaca, Mexico. Indigenous Mazatec shamans employ it for religious purposes and healing, especially for intestinal problems like diarrhea and inflammatory disorders.

HISTORY

It is uncertain how far back in history the use of *Salvia divinorum* extends. Jean Basset Johnson described the plant's role in Mazatec society in the late 1930s. Alfredo Ortega and Leander Valdes III independently isolated salvinorin A in the early 1980s, and Valdes gave it its name. In the 1990s, Daniel Siebert demonstrated the psychoactivity of vaporized pure salvinorin A.

CHEMISTRY/PHARMACOLOGY

Salvinorin A contains no nitrogen atom; that is, it is not an alkaloid. Instead, it is a terpene, a family of substances that are important in the world of fragrances, tastes, and colors. Pure salvinorin A, however, is odorless, tasteless, and colorless.

Salvinorin A also is unique among the compounds in this handbook in that its activity is primarily due to stimulating the kappa-opioid receptor.[36] It has no discernible activity at serotonin and norepinephrine sites. More recent data indicate a role for dopamine and cannabinoid[37] receptors. The results of a small number of brain imaging studies are similar to those with the classical compounds.

DOSE AND ROUTES OF ADMINISTRATION

Salvinorin A is the most potent naturally occurring psychedelic, producing psychological effects at doses not much greater than those for LSD. Vaporized salvinorin A is active at 125–1,000 µg.[38] These doses are so small that one needs an expensive analytical balance to measure them accurately.

Other routes of administration are smoking dried leaves, taking a *Salvia divinorum* extract sublingually, or chewing fresh or dried leaves and allowing for sublingual absorption. One may also fortify any other smokable plant material with extract. If using the extract sublingually, or extract-fortified leaves, it is advisable to start with a very low dose.

---

36. While ibogaine is also active at the kappa receptor, this is only one of several mechanisms by which it exerts its effects.

37. For example, THC (tetrahydrocannabinol) and CBD (cannabidiol).

38. LSD is active at between 50–400 µg.

The chewing-and-sublingual-absorption method requires ten to thirty fresh or dried leaves. One chews them very slowly, keeps them in the mouth for thirty to sixty minutes, and then spits out the used-up plant material. One may also make a tea by crushing twenty to eighty fresh leaves into water.

EFFECTS/SIDE EFFECTS

Effects from the tincture begin in ten to fifteen minutes, peak quickly, and are mostly gone within an hour. The quid (chewing) method produces full effects within a half hour, which continue for another thirty to sixty minutes.

Effects of smoked salvinorin A begin almost instantly, peak at two to five minutes, and are mostly gone within forty-five minutes. However, lingering and disorienting effects may last longer. Higher doses lead to the loss of awareness of external sensory perception, amnesia, and difficulty distinguishing between drug effects and external reality. At lower doses— or with the sublingual or oral routes—a dark room and/or closed eyes may be necessary to discern visual effects, which may be too subtle in a well-lit room or with eyes open.

Changes in body image are common—merging with objects in the environment through physical sensations of stretching, spreading, or dissolving. One may not be able to communicate or move. Entrance into a hallucinatory world wherein one encounters entities or beings may occur.

It may not be possible to distinguish drug effects from what is taking place in the real world and a person under the influence may attempt to interact physically with hallucinated objects. Thus, we might consider salvinorin A to be a "true psychotomimetic" where insight disappears. It is highly advisable that a strong and sober sitter is available to prevent the intoxicated person from injuring themself.

This loss of insight differs from DMT and ketamine, which also provide access to a dissociated world, but where one maintains an awareness that "there is the DMT/ketamine world" and "there is the real world." With salvinorin A, however, one may forget that he or she has taken a drug. Or if they do remember, believe that the drug has changed physical reality. This breakdown in the normal boundaries between reality and the hallucinatory world of salvinorin A is probably responsible for many people never wanting to take it more than once. On the other hand, some find the salvinorin A experience uniquely appealing.

When smoked, salvinorin A does not affect heart rate or blood pressure.

ADVERSE EFFECTS

The intense dissociation and loss of one's ability to distinguish between drug effects and objective reality that may occur with high doses of salvinorin A may lead to flashbacks more frequently than with other psychedelics.

I have found no data indicating that salvinorin A is neurotoxic or causes damage to other organs.

LEGAL

US federal law does not criminalize salvinorin A or *Salvia divinorum*. However, several states have made possession of the plant and/or extracts illegal.

PART IV

PRACTICAL GUIDELINES

CHAPTER 11

HOW TO TRIP

Many of us refer to a psychedelic drug experience as a "trip" or "journey." As with any trip or journey, the more exotic, unfamiliar, and potentially challenging our destination, the more we must do to make sure we are ready. Therefore, I believe it is important to provide guidelines that will help make your experience positive and reduce the risk of a negative outcome.

The three pillars of any psychedelic drug experience are set, setting, and dose. I believe that set—our psychological, physical, and spiritual state, as well as our intention—is the most important leg of this tripod.

Leo Zeff—also known as "the Secret Chief"—was a Bay Area psychologist who died in 1988. Over several decades, he supervised thousands of psychedelic drug experiences. His toolkit included MDMA, LSD, psilocybin, ibogaine, MDA, and ketamine, in addition to eyeshades, comfortable mats, and a wide range of music. I was lucky to have Leo as a mentor in the mid-1980s.

One of Leo's important insights was that simply deciding to take a psychedelic drug meant that "the trip had already begun." Our lives have now come under the "influence" of the drug, and we have started thinking about it. What will the trip be like? How should I prepare? What is the best setting? And what will my life be like afterward?

The suggestions that follow relate to full psychedelic doses of these substances. The effects of smaller doses, as I will describe in the next chapter, are not fully psychedelic and usually do not require as much preparation. Nevertheless, if you are uncertain regarding how any dose of a psychedelic will affect you, these procedures for higher-dose experiences are relevant. These instructions will be helpful, too, if you are raising your "microdoses" to more mega ones and want to be prepared if effects are unexpectedly strong.

LONG-TERM PREPARATION

This is the least psychedelic-specific stage; instead, it has to do with the overall direction your life is taking. Do you orient yourself toward pleasure from the world around you—food, travel, and entertainment? Do spiritual questions take priority? Do you wish to know if there is a Higher Power, God, or angels? Do you wonder about normally invisible worlds that you believe exist but have not experienced firsthand? Creative urges—artistic or scientific—may drive your ambitions in life. Is psychological or emotional knowledge your highest goal—understanding and changing how you feel, think, and behave?

Regardless of why anyone decides to take a psychedelic, remember that these substances are called "psychedelic" for a reason. They are mind manifesting or mind disclosing. In preparation, therefore, it is best to gain some familiarity with your mind no matter what your intention. You may have experiences during any trip that require self-knowledge to successfully navigate. This is an inner voyage, not one that simply requires a passport or plane ticket.

Two broad approaches to self-knowledge, time-tested and reliable, are psychotherapy and spiritual practice. Both approaches require energy, concentration, and commitment to self-examination and change. The differences between the two are not as clear-cut as one might imagine. We see this, for example, in the case of the Anonymous programs where emphasis on a "Higher Power" mixes easily with traditional group and individual psychotherapeutic processes.[39]

The number of present-day religions with at least hundreds of millions of adherents and thousands of years of tradition are few: Judaism, Christianity, and Islam in the West, and Buddhism and Hinduism in the East. They differ in their beliefs, which in turn determine how they attempt to improve our lives. For example, Buddhism teaches that our spiritual development rests entirely in our own hands, as there is no external deity. Thus, their meditation practices emphasize developing self-awareness to bring about mental states that lead to the goal of enlightenment. God-oriented Western religions, on the other hand, include looking outside of ourselves. One attains salvation or blessedness by prayer toward, and works in service of, an external deity. It is similarly important, however, in both Western and Eastern settings to find and work within a community of dependable, empathic, and encouraging peers and teachers. Do your homework and avoid cults or other potentially abusive or dangerous settings. Many religious institutions, even the most mainstream, find it difficult to avoid preying on those who seek their help.

Traditional psychotherapy's goals are more modest, concerned with issues of everyday life.[40] The psychotherapeutic process begins with acknowledging emotional or psychological pain, difficult relationships, or not living up to our potential. Most often, this work occurs in a one-to-one setting but may also involve group therapy. It employs verbal communication or "talk

---

39. The relationship between Anonymous programs and any pharmaceuticals can be complex. Some groups advise complete avoidance of any "psych meds," whereas others are more flexible. And let us not forget how positively Bill Wilson, cofounder of Alcoholics Anonymous, viewed LSD after his own experiences with it in the 1950s.

40. A good psychotherapist will recognize the limits of their own expertise and refer you to a spiritual teacher when religious/spiritual goals become increasingly important. At the same time, a good spiritual teacher will make a psychotherapy referral when psychological problems interfere with one's spiritual growth.

therapy" to access feelings, memories, and thoughts that we normally avoid or are unaware of. By shedding light on them, they control us less.

SHORT-TERM PREPARATION

While the long-term work is that of a lifetime, the suggestions I now present are more psychedelic-specific. They follow your decision to take a trip with one of these substances. They might extend over two to four weeks before your trip, and end only once you have taken the psychedelic drug and the trip itself begins.

I cannot emphasize enough the importance of education. In fact, that is the entire point of this handbook! Some might object to this recommendation and say that studying up on the psychedelic experience will have too much influence on what takes place. This is unreasonable. It is better to be prepared than unprepared. Preparation reduces the risk of being surprised and increases the likelihood that you will recognize, effectively work with, and benefit from what you encounter while tripping.

While everyone's experience is different, there are broadly similar features that nearly everyone encounters on any particular drug—from 5-methoxy-DMT to ibogaine. Through educating ourselves, we can get a general sense of where we are going: the "geography," "climate," even the "inhabitants" and their customs and forms of communication. You do not want to enter such an exotic landscape not knowing what to expect. For example, you should know that a high dose of DMT may cause you to lose awareness of your body—but that does not mean you are dead. Having this foreknowledge will ease your fears when this "loss of the body" takes place. The fully psychedelic experience is often unlike anything else one has ever contended with, and you owe it to yourself to be ready.

Books and other media about these fascinating drugs are more widespread than ever—covering both academic and popular material, as well as first-person accounts. Seek out others who have tripped, listen to talks, join online discussion groups. All will help you to get ready, know better what to expect, navigate your journey successfully, and aid the integration of your trip into daily life.

There also is a vast body of literature on other altered states of consciousness that share features with the psychedelic ones. These include the near-death and out-of-body experiences, meditation and prayer, enlightenment and prophecy, and alien abduction. Familiarity with these psychedelic-like states—how others have interpreted and worked with them—can help you approach, understand, and apply what happens to you when you trip.

If you are in therapy and/or have a spiritual teacher, let them know about your decision to take a psychedelic journey. Do not be surprised, however, if they react with disapproval or discouragement. These reactions may occur because your therapist or teacher does not know about psychedelic drugs, has had unpleasant experiences with them, or may have well-thought-out arguments about why psychedelics are not advisable. Whatever the case, they ought to respect your decision, approach it with curiosity and empathy, and discuss things with you openly. If you face unremitting opposition to your decision, you can forgo your trip, find another teacher/therapist, or keep your experiences to yourself. The last option may involve not telling the whole truth, which is less than ideal.

HEALTH

Remember that psychedelic drugs are chemicals. They change our bodily chemistry, especially that of the brain. Keep things simple and safe by paying extra attention to optimizing your overall health, including medication and substance use. Make certain to coordinate any potential changes in your medication regimen—and if appropriate, share your plans to take a psychedelic—with your healthcare providers, and especially with your prescribers. If you are in poor health, please begin with very low doses of any psychedelic.

Psychiatric drugs may interact with psychedelics in unpredictable ways—increasing, decreasing, or otherwise changing your response to them. If you can successfully stop taking psychiatric medications, it is best to wait a month or two and see how you do without them. This also holds true for excessive substance use, including tobacco, vaping, alcohol, caffeine, cannabis, or cocaine.

Medical conditions for which you take medication may also complicate matters. For example, high blood pressure may get worse during your trip and/or blood pressure medication may not mix safely with a psychedelic. Only if lifestyle changes work as well as medication for conditions like obesity, high blood pressure, or type 2 diabetes, you may then substitute these lifestyle changes for medication and embark on a psychedelic journey more safely.

DECIDING ON DOSE

How much of any psychedelic you take depends on the set and the setting—your mental, spiritual, and physical state; why you are tripping; and in what circumstances. In addition to the medical-biological factors I just addressed, your previous experience with psychedelics also plays a role. The more practice you have had tripping, the more skilled you are in managing both positive and negative effects. If you are ready to explore the effects of higher doses, do not forget that it is not possible to predict the outcome of any particular drug experience, especially at higher doses.

CLARIFYING INTENTION

"Why do I want to take a psychedelic drug?" "What do I hope to gain from my trip?" "What do I wish to avoid?" How we answer these questions is crucial in determining where and with whom we trip, as well as the dose we take. Here are several categories of experiences that most people seek when they take a psychedelic journey.

NEW, UNUSUAL, AND EXCITING EXPERIENCES. Are you curious and seeking novelty? Are you eager to travel through space and time, encounter alternate realities that feel more real than real, even meet their inhabitants? These types of trips require high doses.

PROBLEM-SOLVING. Do you have problems you wish to resolve that you have not been successful resolving in your regular state of consciousness? You may wish to gain new insights about how to deal with creative, professional, psychological, and/or interpersonal obstacles. The mental functions involved in problem-solving are different from those used while traveling through time and space. For this kind of work, you must retain the ability to think, even though your thought processes may take on new power and perspective. You also want to remember the solutions you come up with. Therefore, lower to mid-range doses will loosen sensory, psychological, and creative chains but still allow you to function.

SPIRITUAL GROWTH. Consider the full range of doses in this case, depending on the nature of the experience you seek. For example, lower doses may aid your understanding of spiritual texts; medium doses may enhance prayer or meditation; and higher doses can potentially propel you into the most exalted realms. While we now frequently hear about the mystical-unitive state, this is not the only type of religious experience possible. Psychedelics may be at least as useful for the interactive-relational type I have discussed previously.

GREED, HATE, AND DELUSION. Not everyone takes psychedelics for noble purposes. These three "great poisons" of Buddhism—beliefs and their resulting actions that lead to our own and others' suffering—may motivate you, too. Do you have darker intentions? Is there someone or some group you wish to hurt, abuse, or make money from? Do these darker motives take aim at yourself; that is, to replay abusive past or present relationships solely to increase self-pity and confirm your negative self-image? For example, are you in an abusive relationship and your intention is to empathize with your violent partner, to "understand" them? Here, the healthier motive might be to resolve to leave this partner, rather than bringing yourself closer to your enemy.

There are likely many reasons to take a psychedelic drug. Not all are conscious, and some may conflict with each other. This means that any experience may be quite different from the one for which you planned. An eagerly anticipated mystical experience may instead become one that deals with career issues. A hoped-for journey through inner/outer space may turn out to be quite down to earth and provide an answer to a health-related problem. And of course, the fun trip you wish for may turn out to be painfully difficult.

LAST-MINUTE PLANS

Make certain to take care of as many loose ends as possible before you trip. Tell those to whom you are close about your decision and ask for their advice and support. To the extent possible, clear the air between you and anyone with whom you may be in conflict. And do not forget about paperwork that you would rather not have to think about. While updating your will seems morbid, it may relieve some of your anxiety when you lose awareness of your body and wonder if you have died.

Print a copy of basic rules and follow them during your session, as it may be difficult to remember them while intoxicated. For example, "Don't take higher doses or additional drugs than what I originally planned." "Do not drive until tomorrow." "Drink plenty of water." Have handy the name and phone number of the person who knows you are tripping if you begin to panic.

Decide if you will keep your phone on. Especially with higher doses, the fewer intrusions the better; but at lower doses, you may want to explore interacting with others through your phone while tripping.

SETTING

This section deals with solo trips. Later in this chapter, I turn to the group setting, which is after all, a collection of individual ones.

OUTDOORS OR INDOORS

OUTDOORS. Psychedelics may profoundly enhance nature appreciation; for example, we see for the first time the interconnectedness of all the natural world, including our own place in it. We might ecstatically melt into the ground or merge with a majestic large tree. However, an outdoor setting is less predictable than most indoor ones. Sudden weather changes, insects, unwelcome people or animals, and lack of facilities are all potential complicating factors. Therefore it is advisable to trip outdoors with a non-intoxicated companion. They can help take care of any unforeseen circumstances. And unless there is someone sober with you, I do not advise high doses outdoors.

Tripping in an outdoor urban environment can also provide many new and interesting aesthetic experiences, as well as a deeper understanding of human nature. Think about sightseeing in Times Square in New York City on LSD or mushrooms, or strolling up and down a mammoth indoor mall in suburbia after taking MDMA. Low or medium doses allow you to react appropriately to most situations you may encounter in these settings. Nevertheless, I suggest including a non-intoxicated companion to help you navigate through any unexpected, unpleasant, or frightening encounters.

INDOORS. It is easier to prepare and control indoor spaces, and they are safer and more predictable than outdoor ones. By "indoor," I mean one's home, a therapist's office, or a clinical research suite. Larger indoor venues like a house of worship or retreat center, and especially a massive indoor stadium, are more like urban settings in terms of planning.

An indoor setting is also convenient if you are tripping to do something, rather than simply to have an experience. Here, lower to medium doses make it easier to write, create art, dance or sing, or work on your computer.

While natural beauty can be spectacular, you can make your indoor space equally beautiful on a smaller scale. Prepare your tripping space with care. While under the influence, you will experience thoughts, feelings, and sensations more intensely and meaningfully, so be sure that what is in your indoor space does not conflict with your goals. For example, while contemplating a lifeless plant might lead to valuable reflections on death and dying, most of us would rather gaze at a beautiful healthy one.

Make your indoor space clean, airy, and quiet, especially if you will take a large dose and cannot easily move to another location. This is important if you take a very high dose with the intent of completely dissociating from the outside world. People differ, though, and a less well-organized environment may be just as or more comfortable for some.

There are advantages and disadvantages to both indoor and outdoor settings. The ideal is a combination of both; that is, a comfortable indoor space with easy access—just out the front door if possible—to natural beauty.

MUSIC

It is so easy and convenient to listen to music with earbuds. Before long, augmented reality headsets also will be in common use. Should you supplement your psychedelic experience using these devices? Once again, you should consider set, setting, and dose. The more potentially unpredictable an environment is, the more sense it makes to avoid having to deal with too much input when tripping. If you wish to immerse yourself in technology while tripping on a large dose, you may wish to remain indoors where unexpected interruptions are less likely.

Music plays a significant role in one's psychedelic experiences because of our heightened emotional responses to it. Silence, too, may intensify and direct psychedelic experiences differently from music, and it is worth fitting into any session. Instrumental-only music, or lyrics in a language you do not understand, may evoke a wider range of emotions than those containing lyrics in your everyday language.

Spiritual music—Eastern, Western,[41] or Indigenous—may also affect you powerfully, but in this case, remember that this genre carries information specific to that tradition. All music is a product of a culture and the beliefs that determine it. With religious music, these themes are more explicit, built into the music intentionally. For example, Eastern spiritual music comes from a worldview much different from Jewish or Christian music. And Jewish and Christian music—quite different from each other—evoke feelings consistent with the religion's beliefs.

Prepare a playlist before your session or make your choices during the trip according to your mood. There also are playlists online designed specifically for psychedelic experiences. In either case, do not feel you cannot change what you are listening to. In both individual and group settings, the "one-vote veto" rule is in force. If someone does not like the music, you will honor that person's preference. In the case of a solo trip, that is you!

---

41. "Western world," not "country Western."

EYESHADES

Eyeshades help maintain an inner focus during your trip. I recommend them for very short-acting compounds like DMT, 5-methoxy-DMT, salvinorin A, as well as injected or snorted ketamine. Otherwise, the external world, even a calm and quiet one, can be too distracting. During a longer trip, especially at higher doses, periods of eyeshade use can also deepen your experience.

VISUAL AIDS

During the LSD sessions that Leo Zeff supervised, he reviewed family photos that participants had brought for that purpose—what he called the "picture trip." These images stirred up feelings, memories, and associations that are especially useful for a psychotherapeutic or spiritually oriented session. He also asked participants to gaze at a mirror at some point during the day. This likewise activated an abundance of material to process in the altered state.

Art materials may be especially useful during the coming-down phase, allowing you to reestablish contact with the physical world more creatively.

HEALTH

For short-acting drugs, fasting is advisable. If this is impractical, have a small amount of water, and if you are a coffee addict, your favorite beverage an hour or two beforehand—preferably without sugar or milk. For long-acting drugs, a light meal beforehand will help stave off hunger pangs toward the end of the day. Interestingly, the UDV ayahuasca church recommends eating before sessions so that if vomiting occurs, it is not with an empty stomach. Drink fluids throughout your experience, especially with stimulating substances like MDMA or long-acting ones like LSD and ibogaine. Once most drug effects are gone, do not overdo eating despite your hunger.

Be careful with other mind-altering substances either during your trip or immediately thereafter: alcohol, cocaine, amphetamines, cannabis, tobacco, or caffeine. Experienced marijuana users may find that judicious use of cannabis helps with anxiety or other temporary difficulties during a psychedelic experience. It may also serve as a catalyst for taking the next step in one's session. However, routinely mixing drugs is rarely a good idea, as you will be muddying the psychedelic waters by adding another drug's effects to your already-altered consciousness. Combining drugs can be dangerous medically, too, potentially raising body temperature, blood pressure, or heart rate to dangerously high levels, or producing a confused state.

TRIPPING WITH OTHERS

In a group setting, you now interact with other personalities—multiple sets. This holds true even if not everyone is tripping.

One model of group administration is for each person to have a solo experience, at least until drug effects begin to wear off. Everyone lies on the floor, headphones/earbuds and eyeshades in place. As the session winds down, those who wish to interact leave the main area to do so.

Usually, however, people trip together to share their experiences while under the influence. Combining forces in the psychedelic session, much like the increased energy and focus available in any goal-directed group activity—church, sporting events, or a concert—will intensify and direct your experiences in ways unavailable when journeying by yourself.

Group experiences can partake of all the types of trips we have discussed: aesthetic and pleasure-oriented, problem-solving, spiritual, and psychological. The psychedelic drug effect will amplify and modify how the group experiences any of these activities: playing music or singing, praying or meditating, working on personal or professional problems. In preparing for a group experience, therefore, it is best to make the intention of the group explicit beforehand. "Why are we all here tripping together?" is not something you want to be asking as drug effects begin.

Group settings require attention to additional details. How do you let people know you need help? What type of assistance is available? How do you address problems in the setting; for example, music, smells,[42] lighting, and room temperature. Will everyone be tripping and how will you know? If so, is everyone on the same drug and dose?

Participants should agree to refrain from sexual and/or aggressive behaviors—verbal, emotional, or physical. This is where skilled supervision of drug sessions is extremely important, as you may not know when you have crossed important boundaries. Remember that "no" always means "no," and "yes" may become "no" during the session. However, "no" never becomes "yes" during a drug experience.

Do not ask for or accept favors that extend outside of the session. You might ask for a blanket when cold, or a glass of water when thirsty, but negotiating a loan or gift, or committing to a relationship, is a different matter. Discuss such things after everyone is sober, the next day at the earliest.

Stay at the site of the group until agreed-upon criteria occur; for example, a certain time frame after which drug effects are mostly absent. Driving a car is a particularly important matter. Will you sleep over at the site and drive home the next day, or have someone sober drive you home if you are still under the influence? Do everything possible to ensure your safety.

Sharing with the group as drug effects subside, especially after higher doses, is one of the great advantages of the group setting. It provides an additional avenue through which to reenter normal consciousness, interpret your experiences, and begin the all-important integration process.

---

42. I recommend not wearing strong perfume or cologne in any group setting.

COUPLES

Psychedelic-assisted couples therapy or marital therapy is a "group" experience, although rarely consisting of more than two people. MDMA may be especially useful for this purpose because of its powerful emotional and interpersonal effects. However, low or medium doses of any longer-acting drug—as well as ketamine—are potentially useful in this setting. Psychedelics may help you become more empathic, lower your emotional guard, and communicate more directly. With or without a facilitator—someone who is usually psychotherapeutically trained—the format may follow the group guidelines I just discussed: time alone, and time together addressing relationship issues. Here, the decision to engage sexually is more nuanced and complex. My general recommendation is to keep things nonsexual until the end of the day, as the primary focus of such sessions should be emotional, psychological, and oriented toward improving communication. If, on the other hand, the couple's intentions are primarily aesthetic, fun, pleasure oriented, sex under the influence may be especially novel and gratifying.

THE SITTER

When tripping alone or in a group, you may decide to utilize supervision or leadership from someone else. This is the "sitter." This person, or people, performs many of the same functions as a babysitter—attending to your needs empathically while at the same time gently but firmly maintaining appropriate limits to your behavior. They also address physical needs—providing water, a blanket, comforting touch, and cleaning up any messes you make. "Sitting" also refers to sitting meditation, where one maintains a sense of alert but unobtrusive awareness of what is going on in the environment, and what may be necessary when circumstances require intervention.

With shorter-acting drugs, this finely tuned active-passive balance is especially useful. When undergoing such a brief and intense experience, one needs to feel supported while at the same time free to journey wherever the drug leads free of distractions. With high doses of longer-acting compounds, alone or in a group, sitters are also important. Confusion may reign either within yourself or in the group, and trusted sitters provide needed structure.

There are settings in which those who supervise drug sessions are more active than passive. For example, in shamanic settings, a host of activities play a role in the process: instrumental and vocal music; and physical interventions like laying on of hands, application of various liquids, and blowing smoke onto parts of one's body.

THE SITTER'S SET

While it is important to be careful whom you trip with, who supervises your experience is even more important. Do your homework. Ask questions both of your prospective sitter and those who have worked with them. What is their training: psychological, spiritual, or otherwise? It is usually the sitters who provide the psychedelic substances themselves, so check their sources. Ask about their motivations. Is it for altruism, fame, money, or influence? Beware of potential sitters who refuse to answer what you believe are important questions. They will usually do this by dismissing their relevance because of their "superior" knowledge and experience. Sexual and financial abuse are sadly not uncommon motivations for some sitters. Do not just take their word for it. Search online for additional information about your prospective sitter(s) and you may discover that you should look elsewhere.

Many of us seek psychedelic drug experiences for their spiritual effects. Therefore, consider the religious or spiritual orientation of your sitter. How do their religious beliefs mesh with yours? Such considerations might seem overly cautious but may be quite relevant to how your sitter supervises your session. If they believe one type of experience is superior to another, their suggestions or interventions during your trip will direct you to a state that you are not interested in, or even worse, that you find antithetical to your beliefs. You may feel disrespected, manipulated, or proselytized.

Is your prospective sitter married and/or a parent? Do you want someone supervising your session who lacks valuable life experiences? What is their personal history with psychedelics? Will they be tripping at the same time? Being in a similar state of consciousness may be helpful, but almost always sitters take a lower dose than those they are sitting for. And if the group is large, it is advisable that not all the sitters partake.

THE TRIP

No matter how well prepared you are, you must be ready for anything and everything during your journey, especially at higher doses. Since much of your mental world is habitual and unconscious, you may be surprised at what comes up during your trip. Remember, too, that psychedelic experiences are remarkably varied, even within one session. You may enter and exit many different states during a single experience. And there is no guarantee that the same drug at the same dose will produce the same effects from one session to the other.

Hopefully, our preparation—both long- and short-term—has led you to a relatively healthy, positive, and clear-eyed approach to your impending journey. You know what you want and have set things up to direct the outcome accordingly. At the same time, you have worked to minimize anything that would lead to a negative experience.

With shorter-acting drugs, sit or lie comfortably. If seated, make sure you have room to lie down if you begin losing body awareness. For longer-acting substances, you might continue your normal activities for a little while—reading, housework, listening to music—until you feel the first indication that something is happening. Then sit or lie down if you have taken a high dose and observe the development of effects. Even if you have taken a small dose and wish to remain active, be extra careful in your movements and decision-making.

GETTING STUCK AND MOVING FORWARD

It is critical to recognize the importance of letting go in helping to make one's way through the psychedelic experience. Passing safely through the initial rush of psychedelic drug effects—with both longer-acting drugs and especially with shorter-acting ones—is easier if you possess this tool. In addition, any time during your session you find yourself resisting, holding on, or fighting the flow of experience, letting go benefits you. In nearly every difficult situation, holding on only worsens discomfort.

An important phase is the loss of body awareness that occurs with short-acting tryptamines, salvinorin A, and ketamine. This invariably produces short-lived anxiety at the onset of effects: a "rush" of inner pressure and rapid acceleration—what feels like consciousness racing out of the body.[43] When you are able to let go, giving up resistance to the separation of body and mind becomes effortless.

So, how do you let go?

Especially valuable is working with your breathing. Breath is a useful way to reestablish equanimity during a difficult phase of the drug experience, at the onset or any other time. Slow, rhythmic, deep, conscious breathing both counteracts any anxiety-related shortness of breath and also provides a general calming effect on the nervous system, even if your breathing is normal. Gain familiarity with these methods before your session so they will be easier to work with when you are under the influence. Many

---

43. If you are "certain" that you have died, an approach I took with my DMT volunteers might be helpful. I suggested they could react in one of two ways: "Oh my God, I'm dying, get me out of here!" Or, "I seem to have died. Very interesting. Now what?"

meditations use the breath: counting inhalations and exhalations, or simply paying attention to them going in and out through the nose.

Paying attention to our bodies can help keep us grounded when psychedelic effects feel overwhelming. Relax tense muscles or areas of your body, such as your abdomen. Gentle yoga postures may be useful in dealing with physical discomfort. Try utilizing your breath to "massage" those areas by directing relaxing attention to them.

ASKING FOR HELP

If you find yourself unable to let go, ask for help. This includes your own resources and those available from others.

If alone, talk things through aloud, listen to how your thoughts sound when spoken, see if you can make sense of them or push more deeply into their meaning or where they may lead. You may also try writing down confusing thoughts, and see how they look once removed. Drink tea, water, or fruit juice. Wrap yourself in a blanket. Change the music. Open or close a window or blinds. Feel your feelings without resisting: if you feel like crying, cry; if you want to laugh, laugh; if nauseous, do not suppress vomiting.

Ask for help from your inner teachers, mentors, spiritual guides, angels, or God. In these latter cases, this often means prayer, and if you have memorized meaningful ones ahead of time, they may be quite effective. Some forms of meditation also partake of prayer, especially visualizations of various deities or guides, as does chanting.

Those in the room with you, if you have prepared well, are also at your service. Share any new insights or obstacles, realizations, or questions, but be careful to not substitute talking for feeling. A good sitter will help you make that distinction. Ask to hold the hand of your sitter or friend, or request other nonsexual touch. Massage may be extremely helpful during a psychedelic trip, but the sexual boundaries must be clear. Discuss with your sitter how you feel about touch before the session.

Prolonged, controlled hyperventilation, "holotropic breath work," can help push you through emotional or physical obstacles, but unless you are quite familiar with this technique, I recommend having someone supervise you. Another technique is to physically push against your sitter, or sitters, build up physical tension, and then at a certain point, release it. This may help push through obstacles that otherwise seem insurmountable. However, this requires skillful application—the sitters must know what they are doing.

BEINGS

DMT, ketamine, and salvinorin A often lead to encounters with "beings," as might any high-dose psychedelic. These "entities," no matter how much you may expect or hope to meet them, are nearly always startling. They are "alive," active, possess intelligence and will, and may even be "expecting" you. They may communicate with you—more or less effectively—or simply ignore you while remaining aware of your presence.

In Chapter 4: How Psychedelics Work: The Brain, I offer my understanding of the nature of the beings. My conclusion is generic and hinges off the definition of "psychedelic." That is, these substances reveal or disclose the previously invisible. I do not come down on one side or the other regarding the beings' objective reality. They, as the "imaginative" contents of any psychedelic experience, represent information that we must decipher using the "rational faculty," our "intellect." How then do we relate to the beings?

Appraise them as you might do when encountering any strangers in a strange land. We do not know their culture, language, nor intent. Nevertheless, we can sense whether they are kind or aggressive, mischievous or serious, or if it is, at the moment, unclear.

Once you establish some stability in your interactions with the beings, and have determined their benign nature, you can engage them in pursuit of information, love, or healing. Keep in mind, though, that trips are always in flux, and beings who first appear safe may turn ugly and aggressive, whereas malignant-appearing ones may become less threatening.

Be wary of interacting with entities possessing menacing features such as stingers and fangs. Listen to what they "say," but with skepticism. If they seem to understand your fears, they may be ultimately useful in your trip. Do not allow any beings to force you to accept or do things, or who become angry when you refuse. And by all means, do not conspire with an entity to manipulate or harm anyone.

THE BAD TRIP

Short-lived rough patches are common in most psychedelic experiences. They either pass quickly on their own or respond to any of the interventions I have already discussed. Nearly everyone who is in good mental and physical health, well prepared, takes a reasonable dose, and is in a supportive environment should make it through a psychedelic session feeling good about what they have experienced.

For more intense or prolonged adverse effects, there is a stepwise progression of interventions, from less to more intrusive.

"Talking down" by someone you trust is the first stage—supportive and empathic listening, questioning, and clarification. They will emphasize that whatever you are experiencing is temporary. Decreasing sensory and/or interpersonal stimulation is essential. Nonsexual physical contact such as hand-holding or gentle massage may help reduce the intensity of a potential crisis. If possible, get yourself moving, outside, in the fresh air—with supervision. A thoughtful change in environment can break a vicious cycle of confusion or fear.

There are a handful of "natural" remedies for a bad trip that is not responding to environmental interventions. These include milk, vitamin C, niacin, nicotinamide, and others. None is supported by rigorous clinical research, but may be worth trying before moving on to the "big guns."

Medication is a last resort, and I do not recommend trying this at home. If you are considering a drug-induced end to your trip, medical personnel should be the ones giving it. Minor tranquilizers are first-line—the benzodiazepines like Valium or Klonopin. Sedation is the most common side effect, with the potential for causing low blood pressure and light-headedness. Finally, one should consider the major tranquilizers, or "antipsychotics," like Thorazine, Haldol, olanzapine, or risperidone. Besides producing sedation, these drugs come with a host of unpleasant side effects, including spasms, muscle stiffness, and serious drops in blood pressure. Nevertheless, they may be effective when nothing else is.

Leo Zeff liked to joke about the sitter taking the Valium, not the client, when negative effects seem too intense. In saying this, he reinforced how important are the reactions of those helping someone in distress. The calmer those around someone having difficulties, the calmer that person will be.

THE RESEARCH SETTING

Participating in a research study either as a patient or "normal" volunteer brings together a unique combination of set and setting considerations. The primary difference is the role of altruism. You are not only tripping for yourself, but also for the research and larger communities.

Any type of trip we have discussed may be the subject of a scientific project. Researchers may go to where you are taking a psychedelic—so-called "field research;" for example, during a psychedelic religious ceremony. They may take blood, perform interviews, or have you fill out questionnaires. Or you may go to the researchers themselves, for a biological or therapy study.

Clinical research teams expect you to give them something from your journey—biological specimens, brain waves, filled-out questionnaires, or an interview. In exchange, they provide a carefully monitored environment, skilled personnel, FDA-approved drugs, and legality. The informed-consent process will spell out your responsibilities and rights, as well as what to expect as a research subject. It also should guarantee free treatment for any complications resulting from your participation in the study, and your freedom to withdraw at any point without penalty.

Consider whether your first full psychedelic experience will be in this setting. In some ways, one's first big trip is like sex—perhaps you will be more comfortable as a study volunteer once you have had less constrained and carefully observed experiences. On the other hand, the professional support available in an empathic research setting may make one's first such experience more meaningful and less fraught.

There is less flexibility in the research environment regarding freedom of movement and accoutrements such as music, candles, or incense. While a hospital-based room may feel too clinical, there is the reassuring knowledge that backup is available to manage any unforeseen medical complications.

I suggest learning whether members of the research team have experience with psychedelics, in particular with the drug you will be receiving. Surprisingly, we do not yet have clear-cut answers regarding whether experienced researchers are more effective than inexperienced ones at maximizing positive effects and/or minimizing negative ones. However, it makes sense that those with prior experience will do a better job providing accurate information about what to expect from the drug you will be taking. In addition, if researchers are psychedelic-experienced, they may be more empathic—able to recognize and respond to what you are feeling. In any event, no present-day research studies involve the supervising sitters being on the same drug as you are, so expect every staff member in the room with you to be sober during your experience.

What is the research team's model for the psychedelic experience, their beliefs about it; in other words, the team's set? Their attitude is an essential part of the setting. Do they subscribe to the psychotomimetic model— that psychedelics produce a short-lived form of schizophrenia? If so, prepare for their interactions with you during your trip to reflect these beliefs, interactions that would most likely be different if they believe that psychedelics are mysticomimetic, or are simply pharmacological probes into brain function and consciousness.

If you are in a psychotherapy study, the model is similarly important, perhaps even more so. If a mystical experience is the goal, how does the team react if you "fall short"? And how will that make you feel? And, if a particular experience is the goal of the therapy project, will the team subtly or not so subtly direct your trip in one direction and guide you away from another—even if the one you are now experiencing is thoroughly engaging?

The team may also steer your experience toward a particular goal through their selection of music. Some refer to this half-jokingly as "enlightenment by playlist." However, if your priority is not enlightenment, this playlist may make you unnecessarily uncomfortable. Discuss music with the research team beforehand.

What about the rating scales? Do they emphasize primarily negative effects such as anxiety, fear, confusion, and loss of control as one would expect in a psychotomimetic study; or love, unity, timelessness, and ecstasy in a mysticomimetic one? If you are returning for another session, rating scales will color those subsequent sessions, as you will be looking for those particular effects and not others. Even if there is only one experience with the team, it will affect how you view it afterward during the integration process. Was I insane? Did scores on my questionnaire indicate a "complete" or "incomplete" mystical experience?

INTEGRATION

Integration refers to "what's next?" Now that you have had a big psychedelic experience, what do you do with it? As with preparation, we can divide integration into short-term and long-term processes.

SHORT-TERM

As your experience winds down, you will probably be hungry. Have a light meal and make sure to drink plenty of fluids. Review whatever notes or audio recordings you made. Draw what you saw, especially right after the session. Embellish those images with features reflecting your emotional responses to them. A hot shower or bath may feel wonderful, but avoid raising your body temperature after MDMA, as this drug's toxicity increases with higher body temperatures. Take a nap. Make sure you have nothing pressing to do for the remainder of the day and that night. Take it easy for the next day or two after a big psychedelic experience, especially if it is your first one. Be kind to yourself as you have just returned from a major journey—one that required planning, attention, and mental exertion. A "psychedelic afterglow" may persist for several days or longer after a big trip, so remain open to the process continuing, although at a subtler level, almost behind the scenes.

Make sure to share your experiences with those whom you trust, especially those with whom you shared your intention to trip; for example, friends, mentor, spiritual teacher, or therapist. You do not want to feel isolated, especially if any of the effects were upsetting, disturbing, or difficult to place into the context of your everyday life. If you tripped with a group, you will most likely be sharing your experiences with other participants that day or the next. This is a great opportunity to understand and utilize what happened during your session and to hear about how others dealt with, interpret, and plan to integrate their experiences. If your session occurred in a research setting, there will be a "debriefing" with the research team to answer any questions, provide support, and interpret your experiences within their theoretical framework.

LONG-TERM

Leo Zeff described how the trip "already begins" upon deciding to take a psychedelic journey. Similarly, you have a lot of new material to deal with after a big experience, some of which may extend throughout the rest of your life. That is, "the trip is still happening."

I have already covered much of what is important in long-term integration when discussing long-term preparation. You are the same person you were before your psychedelic journey, but now you have a new benchmark of experience, signposts that are more meaningful than ever. For example, if creative activities are paramount in your life, your trip may have provided new material, conviction, and insight for your work. If you have had doubts about where your life was heading before your session, you may have reached new clarity about the direction you wish to take.

Online forums are helpful. They provide an opportunity to learn about others' experiences as well as to receive support for your own. This kind of peer review offers valuable feedback and makes it less likely that you go off half-cocked onto psychedelic-inspired irresponsible or deluded paths.

You now have the opportunity to align your beliefs and actions with what you felt were the most valuable parts of your session. Engage in activities that remind you of and/or produce the same feelings of truth, beauty, certainty, and goodness. Do not be shy about it if you can do so without harming yourself or others. For example, I have found that studying Hebrew biblical texts evokes many of the feelings and convictions I arrived at during my own formative psychedelic experiences. This seeming change of focus put off some who had been following my work, but allowed me to remain true to the insights I attained during my psychedelic experiences. At the same time, it broadened the range of those interested in my ideas.

If your yoga, meditation, or prayer never felt stronger and more meaningful while tripping, rededicate yourself to these practices and rituals. If you saw solutions to psychological, creative, or professional obstacles, follow through and see how they work. If you felt good and confident about yourself as never before, do not forget that feeling—write it down, think about it, discuss it with important people in your life, and bring it to mind when facing difficult circumstances. If, no matter how many psychedelic sessions you have had, you have made no progress in attaining clarity regarding pressing issues, it may be time to enter psychotherapy rather than taking any more trips.

GETTING HELP

Sharing and peer review serve valuable functions after a good trip. This is even more important if we find ourselves stuck in unshakable distress. These negative outcomes range from anxiety or sadness to depression or psychosis. If you feel on shaky ground, seek help—from the sitter, research team, others with whom you tripped if it was a group experience, therapist, teacher, or loved ones. Such follow-up may range from an hour or two of sharing with a trusted friend all the way to psychiatric hospitalization. While it may be difficult to keep in perspective, remember that you will ultimately benefit from working on and solving the unexpected problems that have come up.

NOW WHAT?

Should we trip again? And when? Why? The answers to these questions vary depending on many of the same issues that led us to take a psychedelic drug in the first place. If we simply wanted help with a specific problem and succeeded, we may not need to trip again. At the other end of the spectrum, our first trip may have initiated us into a spiritual or psychotherapeutic path that involves regular use. In this case, the setting ought to be supervised, safe, and non-cultish. By non-cultish, I mean a group that does not suppress concerns or questions regarding their and their leaders' beliefs and actions.

In between these two poles, we may simply wish to "check in" with ourselves and important people in our lives by periodically taking a psychedelic alone or with others. Once or twice a year, every few years—whatever makes the most sense.

It may take a long time for even one big psychedelic experience to fully exert its effects. Do not get frustrated and seek more drug experiences in order to make the changes in your life you originally expected. Rather, increase your dedication to working on what the first big session showed you.

CHAPTER 12

MICRODOSING

Microdosing refers to taking doses of a psychedelic drug for non-psychedelic effects. Beyond that broad definition, there is little consensus. The practice is increasingly popular, and advocates and enthusiastic media outlets tout its benefits: sharper focus, greater creativity, decreased substance abuse, increased mood, decreased anxiety, better meditation, and increased wellness.

One of the appeals of the microdosing movement is that it removes the stigma of "using drugs," "tripping on mushrooms," or other counterculture antiestablishment behavior. Rather, one is taking something like a vitamin, supplement, or even an antidepressant or stimulant medication. While I understand this approach, it takes the medicalization of psychedelics to an extreme. By treating psychedelics as "super Prozac," one removes the novelty from the psychedelic drug experience. And it is that novelty, the strangeness of the psychedelic state, that draws most of us to these substances. I do not mean to belittle microdosing, but it is important to differentiate between microdosing and having a psychedelic experience.

Here is the title of a scientific study that recently appeared in a prestigious journal: "Adults who microdose psychedelics report health-related motivations and lower levels of anxiety and depression compared to non-microdosers." Sounds great, doesn't it?

The most important principle in evaluating studies like this is: Association does not prove causality. Here is an extreme example that makes this point. Imagine a study reporting that people who exercise are happier than those who do not. Does this mean that exercise causes happiness? Or, that happy people are more likely to exercise than those who are not? In addition, do people who exercise expect that doing so will make them feel better? And when they exercise, do they feel better than those who do not expect to feel better when exercising?

Similarly, do the results of this microdosing study I just referred to mean that microdosing reduces depression and anxiety? Or does it mean that the less depressed and anxious you are, the more likely you are to microdose? In addition, survey studies poll those who expect benefit from microdosing. Why else would they be doing so in the first place? Again, we are dealing with a host of placebo-related factors—expectation, selection bias, and suggestibility.

The science of microdosing is still in its infancy. At the time of this writing (March 2022), there are only about a dozen laboratory studies, and all but one administered only a single microdose rather than multiple doses over time. Since we have so little data, it is not possible to provide definite conclusions or recommendations regarding what microdosing is and what its positive and/or negative effects are.

MICRODOSE DOSES

A common definition of a microdose is one-tenth to one-twentieth of an active dose of a psychedelic drug. However, this is not especially helpful because we need to start with the question: What is an "active dose"? Is it the amount that will give a medium psychedelic experience, an intense one, or a mild one? And sensitivity to psychedelics varies among people, and even within the same person over time. One-tenth of an "active dose" in one person may be a sub-psychedelic microdose, and in someone else it might produce a strong effect. In addition, responses to a microdose may vary from one day to the next.

My approach is to divide microdoses into "tiny," "very small," and "small." And in all cases, we may call these doses "sub-psychedelic." However, this does not mean "sub-psychoactive." I will use examples with LSD, as it comes in more standardized doses than psilocybin-containing mushrooms or DMT-containing ayahuasca.

"Tiny" doses are those that produce no acute subjective effects; i.e., are non-psychoactive. In a laboratory study, volunteers would not be able to distinguish drug from inert placebo, like water or a sugar pill. This might be no more than 5–10 µg of LSD.

"Very small" doses produce noticeable acute effects that are like those of other non-psychedelic drugs; in particular, stimulants like caffeine or methylphenidate (Ritalin). There is an increase in energy, focus, and concentration; a lightening of mood; and more rapid or clear thinking. Ten to twenty µg of LSD would be a "very small" dose.

"Small" doses—greater than 20 µg of LSD—are those that hint at what is to come if one were to increase the dose a little more; for example, subtle perceptual effects such as the room taking on the slightest hint of a sparkle, ideas and associations that are more novel and creative, and a slight sense of anticipation—an inner pressure of expectancy. These are the sorts of effects one feels at the beginning of a full-dose experience.

SUBSTANCES

The most popular microdosing drugs are LSD and psilocybin, especially the latter in the form of dried mushrooms or mushroom tea. Some use low doses of DMT-containing ayahuasca as well as ibogaine. In addition, "stacking" is the practice of adding other substances that theoretically enhance the potential benefit of low doses of classical compounds. These include cacao or chocolate, niacin, and certain medicinal mushrooms. Microdosing ketamine is rare, at least within the model of classical psychedelic microdosing. That is, people take low non-psychedelic doses of ketamine for depression or pain, but not for wellness enhancement.

Neither DMT nor 5-MeO-DMT is orally active, so oral microdosing these compounds will have no pharmacological effect. One could combine either with a monoamine oxidase inhibitor, such as the seeds of Syrian rue, which would produce an ayahuasca-like pharmacology. In addition, the availability of vape pens containing low concentrations of either of these compounds makes feasible microdosing by vaping.

While microdosing MDMA is not as popular as with the classical drugs, it does occur. My concern over neurotoxicity of MDMA disinclines me to recommend microdosing it. All available data, both human and animal, suggest that the more MDMA you take, the more neurotoxicity.

REGIMEN

How often do people microdose? And for how long?

Long-term effects of psychedelic exposure differ from those of acute administration. Early studies of daily low doses of LSD in depressed patients, for example, demonstrated a time course of improvement like what one sees with traditional antidepressants administered daily for several weeks. This is not surprising, as daily LSD dosing produces the same receptor changes in rodent brains as those which occur with the SSRI antidepressants. While tolerance develops to the acute effects of LSD, receptor changes continue evolving and may be responsible for the improvement in mood.

Remember, too, that the psychoplastogenic effects of the classical psychedelics and ketamine occur in animals at non-psychedelic doses after only one administration. These continue for up to a month after exposure, longer in the case of psilocybin than ketamine. This suggests that once per month dosing with psilocybin may be adequate to produce psychoplastogenic changes. And if these changes mediate the effects of microdosing in humans, then monthly dosing may be all that is necessary. Ayahuasca microdosing is a unique case, as it contains MAO-inhibiting compounds similar to prescription antidepressants. Thus, besides the psychoplastogenic effects of DMT, there are additional factors in play due to concurrent effects on MAO.

One may also decide to take a microdose only "as needed," for example, to study before a big exam. In this case, the stimulant-like effects are likely indistinguishable from those of a traditional prescription drug like amphetamine or methylphenidate. The stimulant-like effects of low doses of psychedelics are the subject of a planned study of LSD's effects in ADHD.

In between are schedules that involve taking microdoses on more days than not. Microdose handbooks most frequently advocate this strategy. Here, we are probably seeing a combination of non-psychedelic but psychoactive acute effects, plus longer-term modification of receptor function and psychoplastogenicity. On the other hand, there is little scientific support for this model. Are days off intended to reduce tolerance to the acute psychoactive effects of the drugs? If so, this may require more than simply one or two days of abstinence. In addition, if one finds the acute effects beneficial, wouldn't it make more sense to microdose every day?

RESULTS FROM SURVEYS

Naturalistic online survey studies recruit microdosers and non-microdosers and compare any number of variables between the two groups. Expectancy effects—which contribute to the placebo response—may be as responsible for the positive outcomes as the drugs themselves.[44] That is, if one expects to feel better from microdosing, and then begins doing so, chances are one will feel better. And, if non-psychoactive or non-psychedelic effects enhance the placebo response as I suggested in Chapter 6, this would produce even more substantial effects.

While most reports suggest benefit, not all do. For example, some respondents report increased anxiety and/or depression, insomnia, physical discomfort, headache, fatigue, nausea, overstimulation, and dizziness.

CLINICAL RESEARCH DATA

Laboratory studies of microdosing in humans are only now beginning. The consensus is that single administration of microdoses is doing something— psychological and/or physiological. That is, microdoses are distinguishable from placebo, and subjects describe their effects as "mildly tripping." So, in this case we are dealing with "very small" and "small" doses of drugs, not "tiny" non-psychoactive ones.

Only one study has used a repeated dosing regimen, administering LSD four times at three- to four-day intervals. Neither 13 nor 26 µg doses produced measurable mood or cognition effects. Other research administering only a single microdose of LSD or psilocybin described acute reduction in obsessive-compulsive symptoms, increased feelings of dissociation, variable effects on energy, decreased pain sensitivity, increased creativity, and a speeding up of the subjective passing of time. Low doses of psychedelics may increase or decrease vigilance, concentration, and working memory. In another study, low-dose psilocybin had no effect on emotional processing. Functional brain-imaging research demonstrates that low doses of LSD in normal volunteers increase global connectivity, which appears important

---

44. Expectancy also contributes to the nocebo response, where adverse effects occur from taking an inactive substance.

in the antidepressant response to full doses of psychedelics. Thus, microdoses may be as effective in treating depression as fully psychedelic ones.

CARDIAC EFFECTS?

A theoretical concern of daily use of classical compounds is their potential to damage heart values by chronic stimulation of the serotonin 2B receptor. However, this may be a more theoretical than real concern, since I am unaware of any reports of valvular heart disease in chronic users of ayahuasca, who may drink it several times a week for decades within ayahuasca-using churches and shamanic settings.

CONCLUSIONS

So, is it worth microdosing? Like everything else in this book, one must take stock of the risk-benefit ratio. In the case of microdosing, I believe the risk is low, especially in the case of the oral route of classical psychedelics and ketamine. I say this when it comes to people who do not have any underlying physical or psychiatric conditions, or are taking any medications or other substances, which would make taking a psychedelic drug potentially dangerous. While the "true" benefit may also be low, the "actual" benefit may be higher. That is, placebo effects are real, and to the extent that we can recruit those effects to our advantage, it is worth doing so. Of course, one must do one's homework, do due diligence, know one's source, and be ready to stop and seek help if anything untoward happens.

CHAPTER 13

THE LAW

Neither Ulysses Press nor I advocate taking drugs or breaking the law. Nevertheless, people have taken mind-altering substances—legal and illegal—throughout history. This will not change anytime soon. Therefore, this book is an attempt to educate those who are willing to engage in oftentimes illegal activities. While one might call such an approach "harm reduction," it also partakes of "optimizing benefit."

THE CONTROLLED SUBSTANCES ACT OF 1970

This federal law prohibits illegal importation, manufacture, distribution, possession, and improper use of controlled substances. There are five schedules of controlled substances, with Schedule I being the most restrictive. This is where classical psychedelics, MDMA, and marijuana (!) reside. The criteria are that their abuse potential is high; they have no accepted medical use; and even under medical supervision, lack accepted safety. The US Drug Enforcement Administration (DEA) is responsible for placement of drugs into schedules.

Cocaine, methamphetamine, and fentanyl are in Schedule II, as they possess medical utility—eye anesthesia, ADHD, and pain, respectively. Schedule III drugs are less prone to abuse and have accepted medical use; for example, ketamine for anesthesia. Generic ketamine for depression, however, is "off-label."[45] This means that practitioners may use it for other purposes than anesthesia for which evidence exists regarding efficacy. Patients must give informed consent acknowledging that they are receiving ketamine off-label.

One could argue that current psychedelic research indicates safety under medical supervision, as well as possible medical utility, like therapy for depression, PTSD, and substance abuse. The FDA recognizes this in their designation of MDMA and psilocybin as breakthrough therapies for PTSD and depression, respectively. However, they remain Schedule I drugs under the DEA.

The Controlled Substances Analog Act from the 1990s likewise places into Schedule I compounds that are structurally similar to known Schedule I drugs or have similar effects. Congress passed this law to criminalize "designer drugs" that chemists develop to sidestep prohibitions against known Schedule I compounds. For example, one may add a methyl group here or remove a hydroxy group there from a Schedule I drug, retain the psychedelic effects, but the drug would not appear in the list of scheduled compounds.

The DEA may "emergency schedule" any drug that shows up on their radar that is a candidate for Schedule I placement. After this emergency scheduling, there is a period of public comment, and then the DEA decides whether to formally place it into Schedule I. This is what happened with MDMA in the 1980s. The DEA recently placed several novel tryptamines into Schedule I, one of which is a leading candidate for a commercial psychedelic company's development pipeline.

The law also allows the DEA to carefully monitor and prosecute traffic in "listed chemicals," which are necessary precursors for synthesizing controlled substances. This is the DEA "watch list."

---

45. However, the FDA has approved proprietary Spravato for treatment-resistant depression in combination with ongoing antidepressant therapy.

THE PSYCHEDELIC HANDBOOK

DECRIMINALIZATION AND LEGALIZATION

Participation in approved clinical research studies poses no legal risk, although there remains the stigma of "having tripped on LSD."[46] However, use outside of federally approved research settings for all these drugs in the US is illegal under most municipal and state laws, and all federal ones.

Federal law trumps both state and municipal law, and state law trumps municipal law. This is the most important legal consideration when deciding to take a psychedelic drug. An increasing number of jurisdictions—state, county, and city—have "decriminalized" several aspects of psychedelic substance-related activities. These include growing, synthesizing, possessing, distributing, administering, or consuming such substances. However, the federal DEA may intervene at any time to arrest and prosecute. In addition, states can enforce drug laws despite the enactment of city or county decriminalization.

There are two important concepts that many use interchangeably but which are not identical. These are decriminalization and legalization.

Decriminalization reduces criminal penalties for possession of psychedelics. It may occur in one of two ways. Possession of small amounts of psychedelics for personal, "non-commercial" use is now a civil violation or infraction.[47] However, acquiring psychedelics for personal use remains through illegal markets.

---

46. Or, as the director of the clinical research center in which I performed my DMT and psilocybin studies said one day, "They're smoking mushrooms back there."

47. Civil violations or infractions may carry a fine and/or mandated treatment. Speeding tickets, running a red light, campsite violations, and walking an unleashed dog are examples. One is either responsible or not for civil violations, not innocent or guilty. There may be consequences for civil infractions; say, in the case of a speeding ticket, your insurance rates might increase or you may temporarily lose your license. In general, where possession of small amounts of drugs is an infraction, the infraction does not appear on your criminal record.

Another way decriminalization works is to instruct law enforcement to make combating personal psychedelic use its lowest priority. However, possession of larger-than-permitted quantities for personal use, selling to minors, manufacturing, and distributing remain felonies.[48]

Decriminalization is often the first step toward legalization, which sets into motion more substantial state resources. To date, only Oregon has legalized "psilocybin products." These products include fresh or dried mushrooms, and food or beverages that contain psilocybin mushroom extracts. Those who wish to produce, transport, administer, or sell psychedelics must obtain a state license. Only legalized psychedelic "centers" or "sites of administration" may dispense psilocybin products. Those sites and those who administer the products must meet state certification requirements.[49] California may be the next state to legalize psychedelics. A proposed law legalizes their possession, cultivation, and "sharing."

Psychedelic drug law also varies widely among countries. For example, in the Bahamas it is legal to buy, possess, sell, and use psilocybin and psilocybin-containing mushrooms. In Jamaica, there is no law against psilocybin and psilocybin-containing mushrooms, rather than there being a law allowing their use. In the Netherlands, psilocybin-containing truffles are legal, but not psilocybin-containing mushrooms. In addition, the level of enforcement of international drug laws varies widely.

There is a Talmudic maxim, which I am sure has its equivalent throughout the world: "The law of the land is the law." It is incumbent upon you to familiarize yourself with the legal status of whatever psychedelic substance you intend to consume. And I advise keeping the phone number of an attorney who specializes in drug cases handy in case of trouble.

---

48. A felony is punishable by state prison time. Murder, arson, and rape are felonies. In addition, less severe crimes such as assault and battery with a deadly weapon, and malicious destruction of property over a certain value, are felonies. Long-term consequences of being a "convicted felon" are severe.

49. Oregon has also decriminalized possession of any drug for personal use.

CHAPTER 14

FINAL WORDS

As I began writing *The Psychedelic Handbook*, I thought I was current with the latest research into these extraordinary substances. Even though I had wrapped up my studies at the University of New Mexico in 1995, I have followed the literature, mentored students, given lectures, provided interviews, consulted with academic and pharmaceutical entities, and peer reviewed manuscripts for scientific journals. However, once I started synthesizing the "state-of-the-art," I realized how quickly things have evolved just within the last couple of years. There has been a veritable explosion in academic research, venture capital interest, media attention, and religious debate about the psychedelic drugs.

This book has covered a lot of territory in a short space. Rather than lobby for or oppose the use of psychedelic drugs, my purpose has been to educate—to provide information about these remarkable substances to those who are seeking a balanced introduction by an expert in the field. If I have succeeded, you now have enough information to know what questions to ask if you wish to take your studies further.

It has also been my aim to bring up to date those with a previous background in the world of psychedelics by reviewing the dominant biological and psychological models for their effects. Perhaps as a result, some readers will devise their own scientific experiments!

People take psychedelic drugs. The more they know about what they are taking and how to take them, the fewer problems they will encounter.

Just as important, they may experience more benefits. While much of the scientific information I have presented is drug specific, my intention has also been to teach general principles relevant to all psychedelic drug experiences. That is, besides the drug and its dose, the set and setting within which one takes a psychedelic drug ultimately determines its effects.

It is an extraordinary challenge to understand and study consciousness—the mind, the brain, and the spirit. Psychedelics once held great promise to help answer some of our deepest questions—why we think, act, and feel the way we do; the nature of creativity, dreams, madness, spiritual experience, and death; even the fabric of reality itself. Now, after a generation of neglect, we once again have these powerful "mind-disclosing" tools available to help address these questions. I believe we have learned from the mistakes we made during the first wave of psychedelic enthusiasm, and I look forward to a long, productive era of studying and applying their effects for the common good.

RECOMMENDED READING

CHAPTER 1. WHAT ARE PSYCHEDELICS?

Grinspoon, L., and Bakalar, J. B. (1979). *Psychedelic Drugs Reconsidered*. New York: Basic Books.

Huxley, A. (2009). *The Doors of Perception and Heaven and Hell*. New York: HarperPerennial Modern Classics.

Lee, M. A., and Shlain, B. (1986). *Acid Dreams: The Complete Social History of LSD, the CIA, the Sixties, and Beyond (Revised)*. New York: Grove Press.

Lewin, L. (1998). *Phantastica: A Classic Survey on the Use and Abuse of Mind-Altering Plants*. Rochester, Vermont: Inner Traditions/Bear & Co.

McQueen, D. (2021). *Psychedelic Cannabis. Breaking the Gate*. Rochester, Vermont: Inner Traditions/Bear & Co.

Pollan, M. (2018). *How to Change Your Mind. What the New Science of Psychedelics Teaches Us about Consciousness, Dying, Addiction, Depression, and Transcendence*. New York: Penguin Press.

Rätsch, C. (2005). *The Encyclopedia of Psychoactive Plants*. Rochester, Vermont: Park Street Press.

Schultes, R. E., Hofmann, A., and Rätsch, C. (1998). *Plants of the Gods*. Rochester, Vermont: Healing Arts Press.

Stafford, P. (2013). *Psychedelics Encyclopedia*. Berkley, California: Ronin Publishing.

Stevens, J. (1998). *Storming Heaven: LSD and the American Dream*. New York: Grove Press.

CHAPTER 2. THE MANY NAMES FOR PSYCHEDELICS: WHY THEY MATTER

Gerber, D. J., and Tonegawa, S. (2004). "Psychotomimetic Effects of Drugs—A Common Pathway to Schizophrenia?" *New England Journal of Medicine*, 350, 1047–1048.

Gillin, J. C., Kaplan, J., Stillman, R., and Wyatt, R. J. (1976). "The Psychedelic Model of Schizophrenia: The Case of N,N-dimethyltryptamine." *American Journal of Psychiatry*, 133, 203–208.

Hollister, L. (1962). "Drug-Induced Psychoses and Schizophrenic Reactions: A Critical Comparison." *Annals of the New York Academy of Science*, 96, 80–92.

James, W. (1991). *The Varieties of Religious Experience*. New York: Triumph Books.

Lahti, A. C., Weiler, M. A., Tamara, M., Parwani, A., and Tamminga, C. A. (2001). "Effects of Ketamine in Normal and Schizophrenic Volunteers." *Neuropsychopharmacology*, 25(4), 455–467. doi: 10.1016/S0893-133X(01)00243-3.

Richards, W. A. (2016). *Sacred Knowledge. Psychedelics and Religious Experiences*. New York: Columbia University Press.

Vardy, M. M., and Kay, S. F. (1983). "LSD Psychosis or LSD-Induced Schizophrenia? A Multi-Method Inquiry." *Archives of General Psychiatry*, 40, 877–883.

Sanz, C., and Tagliazucchi, E. (2018). "The Experience Elicited by Hallucinogens Presents the Highest Similarity to Dreaming within a Large Database of Psychoactive Substance Reports." *Frontiers in Neuroscience*, 12(7). doi: 10.3389/fnins.2018.00007.

CHAPTER 3. WHAT ARE PSYCHEDELICS GOOD FOR? WHAT ARE THEIR RISKS?

Benefits

Bogenschutz, M. P., Forcehimes, A. A., Pommy, J. A., Wilcox, C. E., Barbosa, P. C. R., and Strassman, R. J. (2015). "Psilocybin-assisted Treatment for Alcohol Dependence: A Proof-of-Concept Study." *Journal of Psychopharmacology,* 29(3), 289–299. doi: 10.1177/0269881114565144.

Carhart-Harris, R., Giribaldi, B., Watts, R., Baker-Jones, M., Murphy-Beiner, A., Murphy, R., . . . Nutt, D. J. (2021). "Trial of Psilocybin versus Escitalopram for Depression." *New England Journal of Medicine,* 384(15), 1402–1411. doi: 10.1056/NEJMoa2032994.

Griffiths, R. R., Johnson, M. W., Carducci, M. A., Umbricht, A., Richards, W. A., Richards, B. D., . . . Klinedinst, M. A. (2016). "Psilocybin Produces Substantial and Sustained Decreases in Depression and Anxiety in Patients with Life-Threatening Cancer: A Randomized Double-Blind Trial." *Journal of Psychopharmacology,* 30(12), 1181–1197. doi: 10.1177/0269881116675513.

Harman, W. W., McKim, R. H., Mogar, R. E., Fadiman, J., and Stolaroff, M. J. (1966). "Psychedelic Agents in Creative Problem Solving: A Pilot Study." *Psychological Reports,* 19, 211–227. doi: 10.2466%2Fpr0.1966.19.1.211.

Jiménez-Garrido, D. F., Gómez-Sousa, M., Ona, G., Dos Santos, R. G., Hallak, J. E. C., Alcázar-Córcoles, M. Á., and Bouso, J. C. (2020). "Effects of Ayahuasca on Mental Health and Quality of Life in Naïve Users: A Longitudinal and Cross-Sectional Study Combination." *Scientific Reports,* 10(1), 4075. doi: 10.1038/s41598-020-61169-x.

Johnson, M. W., Garcia-Romeu, A., Cosimano, M. P., and Griffiths, R. R. (2014). "Pilot Study of the 5-HT2AR Agonist Psilocybin in the Treatment of Tobacco Addiction." *Journal of Psychopharmacology,* 28(11), 983–992. doi: 10.1177/026988111458296.

Reiff, C. M., Richman, E. E., Nemeroff, C. B., Carpenter, L. L., Widge, A. S., Rodriguez, C. I., . . . McDonald, W. M. (2020). "Psychedelics and Psychedelic-Assisted Psychotherapy." *American Journal of Psychiatry, 177*(5), 391–410. doi: 10.1176/appi.ajp.2019.19010035.

Ross, S., Bossis, A., Guss, J., Agin-Liebes, G., Malone, T., Cohen, B., . . . Schmidt, B. L. (2016). "Rapid and Sustained Symptom Reduction Following Psilocybin Treatment for Anxiety and Depression in Patients with Life-Threatening Cancer: A Randomized Controlled Trial." *Journal of Psychopharmacology, 30*(12), 1165–1180.

Risks

Gable, R. S. (1993). "Toward a Comparative Overview of Dependence Potential and Acute Toxicity of Psychoactive Substances Used Nonmedically." *American Journal of Drug and Alcohol Abuse, 19,* 263–281.

Gómez-Sousa, M., Jiménez-Garrido, D. F., Ona, G., Dos Santos, R. G., Hallak, J. E. C., Alcázar-Córcoles, M. Á., and Bouso, J. C. (2021). "Acute Psychological Adverse Reactions in First-Time Ritual Ayahuasca Users: A Prospective Case Series." *Journal of Clinical Psychopharmacology.* doi: 10.1097/jcp.0000000000001343.

Hall, W. (2021). "Ending the Silence around Psychedelic Therapy Abuse." Mad in America. Retrieved from Mad in America website: https://www.madinamerica.com/2021/09/ending-silence-psychedelic-therapy-abuse.

Halpern, J. H., and Pope, H. G., Jr. (2003). "Hallucinogen Persisting Perception Disorder: What Do We Know After 50 years?" *Drug and Alcohol Dependence, 69,* 109–119.

Malcolm, B., and Thomas, K. (2021). "Serotonin Toxicity of Serotonergic Psychedelics." *Psychopharmacology.* doi: 10.1007/s00213-021-05876-x.

Müller, F., Kraus, E., Holze, F., Becker, A., Ley, L., Schmid, Y., . . . Borgwardt, S. (2022). "Flashback Phenomena after Administration of

LSD and Psilocybin in Controlled Studies with Healthy Participants."
Psychopharmacology. doi: 10.1007/s00213-022-06066-z.

Strassman, R. J. (1984). "Adverse Reactions to Psychedelic Drugs. A
Review of the Literature." *Journal of Nervous and Mental Disease*, 172,
577–595.

CHAPTER 4. HOW PSYCHEDELICS WORK: THE BRAIN

Carhart-Harris, R. L., and Friston, K. J. (2019). "REBUS and the
Anarchic Brain: Toward a Unified Model of the Brain Action of
Psychedelics." *Pharmacological Reviews*, 71, 316–344. doi: 0.1124/pr
.118.017160.

da Silva, M. G., Daros, G. C., and de Bitencourt, R. M. (2020). "Anti-
Inflammatory Activity of Ayahuasca: Therapeutical Implications in
Neurological and Psychiatric Diseases." *Behavioural Brain Research*. doi:
10.1016/j.bbr.2020.113003.

Nichols, D. E. (2016). "Psychedelics." *Pharmacological Reviews*, 68,
264–355.

Olson, D. E. (2022). "Biochemical Mechanisms Underlying Psychedelic-
Induced Neuroplasticity." *Biochemistry*. doi: 10.1021/acs.biochem
.1c00812.

Saeger, H. N., and Olson, D. E. "Psychedelic-Inspired Approaches for
Treating Neurodegenerative Disorders." *Journal of Neurochemistry*, 19.
doi: 10.1111/jnc.15544.

Vollenweider, F. X., and Smallridge, J. W. (2022). "Classic Psychedelic
Drugs: Update on Biological Mechanisms." *Pharmacopsychiatry*. doi:
10.1055/a-1721-2914.

CHAPTER 5. HOW PSYCHEDELICS WORK: THE MIND

Das, L. S. (1995). *The Facts of Life from a Buddhist Perspective, the Three Trainings, Four Noble Truths, Five Skandhas, Six Perfections, Eightfold Path, and More.* Cambridge, Massachusetts: Dzogchen Publications.

Hall, C. S. (2016). *A Primer of Freudian Psychology.* New York: Plume.

Savage, C. (1955). "Variations in Ego Feeling Induced by D-Lysergic Acid Diethylamide (LSD-25)." *Psychoanalytic Review*, 41, 1–16.

Strassman, R. (2014). *DMT and the Soul of Prophecy.* Rochester, Vermont: Park Street Press.

CHAPTER 6. PSYCHEDELICS, PANACEAS, PLACEBOS, AND PSYCHOPLASTOGENS

Carhart-Harris, R. L., Kaelen, M., Whalley, M. G., Bolstridge, M., Feilding, A., and Nutt, D. J. (2014). "LSD Enhances Suggestibility in Healthy Volunteers." *Psychopharmacology*, 232(4), 785–794. doi: 10.1007/s00213-014-3714-z.

Dupuis, D. (2021). "Psychedelics as Tools for Belief Transmission. Set, Setting, Suggestibility, and Persuasion in the Ritual Use of Hallucinogens." *Frontiers in Psychology*, 12(5486). doi: 10.3389/fpsyg.2021.730031.

Hartogsohn, I. (2018). "The Meaning Enhancing Properties of Psychedelics and Their Mediator Role in Psychedelic Therapy, Spirituality, and Creativity." *Frontiers in Neuroscience*, 12(129). doi: 10.3389/fnins.2018.00129.

Levine, J., and Ludwig, A. M. (1965). "Alterations in Consciousness Produced by Combinations of LSD, Hypnosis, and Psychotherapy." *Psychopharmacologia*, 7, 123–137.

Olson, J., Suissa-Rocheleau, L., Lifshitz, M., Raz, A., and Veissiere, S. (2020). "Tripping on Nothing: Placebo Psychedelics and Contextual Factors." *Psychopharmacology*. doi: 10.1007/s00213-020-05464-5.

Shapiro, A. K., and Shapiro, E. (2000). *The Powerful Placebo: From Ancient Priest to Modern Physician*. Baltimore, Maryland: Johns Hopkins University Press.

CHAPTER 7. CLASSICAL PSYCHEDELICS

Basedow, L. A., Riemer, T. G., Reiche, S., Kreutz, R., and Majić, T. (2021). "Neuropsychological Functioning in Users of Serotonergic Psychedelics–A Systematic Review and Meta-Analysis." *Frontiers in Pharmacology*, 2516. doi: 10.3389/fphar.2021.739966.

Bender, D., and Hellerstein, D. J. (2022). "Assessing the Risk–Benefit Profile of Classical Psychedelics: A Clinical Review of Second-Wave Psychedelic Research." *Psychopharmacology*. doi: 10.1007/s00213 -021-06049-6.

Hoffer, A., and Osmond, H. (1967). *The Hallucinogens*. New York: Academic Press.

Mescaline, Peyote, and San Pedro

Albaugh, B. J., and Anderson, P. O. (1974). "Peyote in the Treatment of Alcoholism Among American Indians." *American Journal of Psychiatry*, 131, 1247–1251.

Dobkin, M. (1968). "Trichocereus Pachanoi: A Mescaline Cactus Used in Folk Healing in Peru." *Economic Botany*, 22(2), 191–194.

Halpern, J. H., Sherwood, A. R., Passie, T., Blackwell, K. C., and Ruttenber, A. J. (2008). "Evidence of Health and Safety in American Members of a Religion Who Use a Hallucinogenic Sacrament." *Medical Science Monitor*, 14, SR15-SR22.

Jay, M. (2019). *Mescaline: A Global History of the First Psychedelic*. New Haven, Connecticut: Yale University Press.

Klüver, H. (1928). *Mescal, and Mechanisms of Hallucinations*. Chicago: University of Chicago Press.

La Barre, W. (1989). *The Peyote Cult* (5th ed.). Norman, Oklahoma: University of Oklahoma Press.

LSD

Carhart-Harris, R. L., Muthukumaraswamy, S., Roseman, L., Kaelen, M., Droog, W., Murphy, K., . . . Nutt, D. J. (2016). "Neural Correlates of the LSD Experience Revealed by Multimodal Neuroimaging." *Proceedings of the National Academy of Sciences*, 113(17), 4853–4858. doi: 10.1073/pnas.1518377113.

Dishotsky, N. I., Loughman, W. D., Mogar, R. E., and Lipscomb, W. R. (1971). "LSD and Genetic Damage." *Science*, 172, 431–440.

Grof, S. (2008). *LSD Psychotherapy* (4th ed.). San Jose, California: Multidisciplinary Association for Psychedelic Studies.

Hofmann, A. (1980). *LSD: My Problem Child*. New York: McGraw Hill.

Liechti, M. E. (2017). "Modern Clinical Research on LSD." *Neuropsychopharmacology*, 42(11), 2114–2127.

Pahnke, W. N., Kurland, A. A., Unger, S., Savage, C., and Grof, S. (1970). "The Experimental Use of Psychedelic (LSD) Psychotherapy." *Journal of the American Medical Association*, 212, 1856–1863.

Wasson, R. G., Hofmann, A., and Ruck, C. A. P. (2008). *The Road to Eleusis: Unveiling the Secret of the Mysteries*. Berkeley, California: North Atlantic Books.

Psilocybin

Anderson, B. T., Danforth, A., Daroff, P. R., Stauffer, C., Ekman, E., Agin-Liebes, G., . . . Woolley, J. (2020). "Psilocybin-Assisted Group Therapy for Demoralized Older Long-Term AIDS Survivor Men: An Open-Label Safety and Feasibility Pilot Study." *EClinicalMedicine*, 11. doi: 10.1016/j.eclinm.2020.100538.

Haze, V., and Mandrake, K. (2016). *The Psilocybin Mushroom Bible: The Definitive Guide to Growing and Using Magic Mushrooms*. San Francisco, California: Green Candy Press.

Kargbo, R. (2020). "Psilocybin Therapeutic Research: The Present and Future Paradigm." *ACS Medicinal Chemistry Letters*, 11, 399–402. doi: 10.1021/acsmedchemlett.0c00048

Smigielski, L., Scheidegger, M., Kometer, M., and Vollenweider, F. X. (2019). "Psilocybin-Assisted Mindfulness Training Modulate Self-Consciousness and Brain Default Mode Network Connectivity with Lasting Effects." *NeuroImage*, 207–215. doi: 10.1016/J.neuroimage .2019.04.009.

DMT/Ayahuasca

Almeida, C. A. F., Pereira-Junior, A. A., Rangel, J. G., Pereira, B. P., Costa, K. C. M., Bruno, V., . . . Camarini, R. (2022). Ayahuasca, a Psychedelic Beverage, Modulates Neuroplasticity Induced by Ethanol in Mice. *Behavioural Brain Research,* 416, 9. doi: 10.1016/j.bbr.2021 .113546.

Barker, S. A. (2022). "Administration of N,N-Dimethyltryptamine (DMT) in Psychedelic Therapeutics and Research and the Study of Endogenous DMT." *Psychopharmacology*. doi: 10.1007/s00213-022-06065-0.

Lawn, W., Hallak, J. E., Crippa, J. A., Dos Santos, R., Porffy, L., Barratt, M. J., . . . Morgan, C. J. A. (2017). "Well-Being, Problematic Alcohol Consumption and Acute Subjective Drug Effects in Past-Year Ayahuasca Users: a Large, International, Self-Selecting Online Survey." *Scientific Reports,* 7(1), 15201. doi: 10.1038/s41598-017-14700-6.

Morales-Garcia, J. A., Calleja-Conde, J., Lopez-Moreno, J. A., Alonso-Gil, S., Sanz-SanCristobal, M., Riba, J., and Perez-Castillo, A. (2020). "N,N-Dimethyltryptamine Compound found in the Hallucinogenic Tea Ayahuasca, Regulates Adult Neurogenesis in Vitro and in Vivo." *Translational Psychiatry*, 10(1), 331. doi: 10.1038/ s41398-020-01011-0.

Nardai, S., László, M., Szabó, A., Alpár, A., Hanics, J., Zahola, P., . . . Nagy, Z. (2020). "N,N-Dimethyltryptamine Reduces Infarct Size and Improves Functional Recovery Following Transient Focal Brain Ischemia in Rats." *Experimental Neurology*. doi: 10.1016/j.expneurol .2020.113245.

Palhano-Fontes, F., Barreto, D., Onias, H., Andrade, K. C., Novaes, M. M., Pessoa, J. A., . . . Araújo, D. B. (2018). "Rapid Antidepressant Effects of the Psychedelic Ayahuasca in Treatment-Resistant Depression: A Randomized Placebo-Controlled Trial." *Psychological Medicine*, 1–9. doi: 10.1017/S0033291718001356.

Strassman, R. J., and Qualls, C. R. (1994). "Dose-Response Study of N,N-Dimethyltryptamine in Humans. I: Neuroendocrine, Autonomic, and Cardiovascular Effects." *Archives of General Psychiatry*, 51, 85–97.

Strassman, R. J., Qualls, C. R., Uhlenhuth, E. H., and Kellner, R. (1994). "Dose-Response Study of N,N-Dimethyltryptamine in Humans. II: Subjective Effects and Preliminary Results of a New Rating Scale." *Archives of General Psychiatry*, 51, 98–108.

Strassman, R. (2001). *DMT: The Spirit Molecule*. Rochester, Vermont: Park Street Press.

5-Methoxy-DMT

Davis, W., and Weil, A. T. (1992). "Identity of a New World Psychoactive Toad." *Ancient Mesoamerica*, 3(1), 51–59.

Most, A. (1984). *Bufo Alvarius: the Psychedelic Toad of the Sonoran Desert*. Denton, Texas: Venom Press.

Reckweg, J. T., Uthaug, M. V., Szabo, A., Davis, A. K., Lancelotta, R., Mason, N. L., and Ramaekers, J. G. (2022). "The Clinical Pharmacology and Potential Therapeutic Applications of 5-Methoxy-N,N-Dmethyltryptamine (5-MeO-DMT)." *Journal of Neurochemistry*, n/a(n/a). doi: 10.1111/jnc.15587.

Uthaug, M., Lancelotta, R., Bernal, A., Davis, A., and Ramaekers, J. (2020). "A Comparison of Reactivation Experiences Following Vaporization and Intramuscular Injection (IM) of Synthetic 5-Methoxy-N,N-Dimethyltryptamine (5-MeO-DMT) in a Naturalistic Setting." *Journal of Psychedelic Studies*, 1–10. doi: 10.1556/2054 .2020.00123.

Ibogaine

Brett, D. (2021). *Iboga: The Root of All Healing*: Noble Sapien.

Fernandez, J. W. (1982). *Bwiti. An Ethnography of the Religious Imagination in Africa*. Princeton, New Jersey: Princeton University Press.

Köck, P., Frölich, K., Walter, M., Lang, U., and Dürsteler, K. M. (2021). "A Systematic Literature Review of Clinical Trials and Therapeutic Applications of Ibogaine." *Journal of Substance Abuse Treatment*, 108717. doi: 10.1016/j.jsat.2021.108717.

Mash, D. C., Duque, L., Page, B., and Allen-Ferdinand, K. (2018). "Ibogaine Detoxification Transitions Opioid and Cocaine Abusers Between Dependence and Abstinence: Clinical Observations and Treatment Outcomes." *Frontiers in Pharmacology*, 9(529). doi: 10.3389/fphar.2018.00529.

CHAPTER 8. MDMA

Costa, G., and Gołembiowska, K. (2022). "Neurotoxicity of MDMA: Main Effects and Mechanisms." *Experimental Neurology*, 347, 113894. doi: 10.1016/j.expneurol.2021.113894.

Holland, J. (2001). *Ecstasy: The Complete Guide: A Comprehensive Look At The Risks And Benefits Of MDMA*. Rochester, Vermont: Inner Traditions/Bear & Co.

Mitchell, J. M., Bogenschutz, M., Lilienstein, A., Harrison, C., Kleiman, S., Parker-Guilbert, K., . . . Doblin, R. (2021). "MDMA-Assisted Therapy for Severe PTSD: a Randomized, Double-Blind, Placebo-Controlled Phase 3 Study." *Nature Medicine*, 27(6), 1025–1033. doi: 10.1038/s41591-021-01336-3.

Montgomery, C., and Roberts, C. A. (2022). "Neurological and Cognitive Alterations Induced by MDMA in Humans." *Experimental Neurology*, 347, 113888. doi: 10.1016/j.expneurol.2021.113888.

CHAPTER 9. KETAMINE

Dillon, P., Copeland, J., and Jansen, K. (2003). "Patterns of Use and Harms Associated with Non-Medical Ketamine Use." *Drug and Alcohol Dependence*, 69(1), 23–28. doi: 10.1016/S0376-8716(02)00243-0.

Horowitz, M., and Moncrieff, J. (2021). "Esketamine: Uncertain Safety and Efficacy Data in Depression." *The British Journal of Psychiatry*, 219(5), 621–622. doi: 10.1192/bjp.2021.163.

Jansen, K. L. R. (2001). *Ketamine: Dreams and Realities*. Sarasota, Florida: Multidisciplinary Association for Psychedelic Studies.

McInnes, L. A., Qian, J. J., Gargeya, R. S., DeBattista, C., and Heifets, B. D. (2022). "A Retrospective Analysis of Ketamine Intravenous Therapy for Depression in Real-World Care Settings." *Journal of Affective Disorders*. doi: 10.1016/j.jad.2021.12.097.

McIntyre, R. S., Rosenblat, J. D., Nemeroff, C. B., Sanacora, G., Murrough, J. W., Berk, M., . . . Ho, R. (2021). "Synthesizing the Evidence for Ketamine and Esketamine in Treatment-Resistant Depression: An International Expert Opinion on the Available Evidence and Implementation." *American Journal of Psychiatry*, 178(5), 383–399. doi: 10.1176/appi.ajp.2020.20081251.

Muetzelfeldt, L., Kamboj, S. K., Rees, H., Taylor, J., Morgan, C. J., and Curran, H. V. (2008). "Journey Through the K-Hole: Phenomenological Aspects of Ketamine Use." *Drug and Alcohol Dependence*, 95(3), 219–229. doi: 10.1016/j.drugalcdep.2008.01.024.

Witt, E. (2021). "Ketamine Therapy Is Going Mainstream. Are We Ready?" *New Yorker*, 17. Retrieved from NewYorker.com website: https://www.newyorker.com/culture/annals-of-inquiry/ketamine-therapy-is-going-mainstream-are-we-ready.

Wolfson, P., and Hartelius, G. (2016). *The Ketamine Papers: Science, Therapy, and Transformation*. San Jose, California: Multidisciplinary Association for Psychedelic Studies.

Zanos, P., Moaddel, R., Morris, P. J., Riggs, L. M., Highland, J. N., Georgiou, P., . . . Zarate, C. A. (2018). "Ketamine and Ketamine

Metabolite Pharmacology: Insights into Therapeutic Mechanisms." *Pharmacological Reviews*, 70(3), 621–660.

CHAPTER 10. SALVIA DIVINORUM/ SALVINORIN A

Doss, M. K., May, D. G., Johnson, M. W., Clifton, J. M., Hedrick, S. L., Prisinzano, T. E., . . . Barrett, F. S. (2020). "The Acute Effects of the Atypical Dissociative Hallucinogen Salvinorin A on Functional Connectivity in the Human Brain." *Scientific Reports*, 10(1), 16392. doi: 10.1038/s41598-020-73216-8.

Ranganathan, M., Schnakenberg, A., Skosnik, P. D., Cohen, B. M., Pittman, B., Sewell, R. A., and D'Souza, D. C. (2012). "Dose-Related Behavioral, Subjective, Endocrine, and Psychophysiological Effects of the κ Opioid Agonist Salvinorin A in Humans." *Biological Psychiatry*, 72, 871–879.

Roth, B. L., Baner, K., Westkaemper, R., Siebert, D., Rice, K. C., Steinberg, S., . . . Rothman, R. B. (2002). "Salvinorin A: a Potent Naturally Occurring Non-Nitrogenous Kappa Opioid Selective Agonist." *Proceedings of the National Academy of Sciences USA*, 99, 11934–11939.

CHAPTER 11. HOW TO TRIP

Gearin, A. K. (2022). "Primitivist Medicine and Capitalist Anxieties in Ayahuasca Tourism Peru." *Journal of the Royal Anthropological Institute*, 20.

Peluso, D. D., Sinclair, E., Labate, B., and Cavnar, C. (2022). "Guidelines Creating Awareness on Sexual Abuse in Ayahuasca Communities: A review of Chacruna's Guidelines." Chacruna. Retrieved from Chacruna.net website: https://chacruna.net/creating-awareness-on-sexual-abuse-in-ayahuasca-communities-a-review-of-chacrunas-guidelines/.

Stolaroff, M. J. (1997). *The Secret Chief: Conversations With a Pioneer of the Underground Psychedelic Therapy Movement*. Santa Cruz, California: The Multidisciplinary Association for Psychedelic Studies.

CHAPTER 12. MICRODOSING

de Wit, H., Molla, H. M., Bershad, A., Bremmer, M., and Lee, R. "Repeated Low Doses Of LSD in Healthy Adults: A Placebo-Controlled, Dose–Response Study." *Addiction Biology*, n/a(n/a), e13143. doi: 10.1111/adb.13143.

Fadiman, J. (2011). *The Psychedelic Explorer's Guide*. Rochester, Vermont: Park Street Press.

Polito, V., and Liknaitzky, P. 2021. "The Emerging Science of Microdosing: A Systematic Review of Research on Low Dose Psychedelics (1955–2021)." PsyArXiv. December 15. doi:10.31234/osf.io/edhqz.

Rootman, J. M., Kryskow, P., Harvey, K., Stamets, P., Santos-Brault, E., Kuypers, K. P., . . . Walsh, Z. (2021). "Adults Who Microdose Psychedelics Report Health Related Motivations and Lower Levels of Anxiety and Depression Compared to Non-Microdosers." *Scientific Reports*, 11(1), 22479. doi: 10.1038/s41598-021-01811-4.

CHAPTER 13. THE LAW

Lampe, J. R. (2021). "The Controlled Substances Act (CSA): A Legal Overview for the 117th Congress." Retrieved from Congressional Research Service website: https://crsreports.congress.gov/product/pdf/R/R45948.

CHAPTER 14. FINAL WORDS

Love, S. (2021). "The False Promise of Psychedelic Utopia." VICE. Retrieved from Vice website: https://www.vice.com/en/article/dypzxj/the-false-promise-of-psychedelic-utopia.

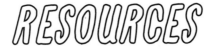

RESOURCES

Beckley Foundation

Supports psychedelic research to drive evidence-based drug policy reform.

Website: beckleyfoundation.org

Blossom Analysis

Weekly newsletter that lists and analyzes scientific and lay literature on the developing field of psychedelics as medicine.

Website: blossomanalysis.com

Clinicaltrials.gov

A database of privately and publicly funded clinical studies conducted around the world.

Website: clinicaltrials.gov

Heffter Research Institute

Designs, reviews, and funds psychedelic research for treatment of addictions and other mental disorders.

Website: heffter.org

Intercollegiate Psychedelics Network

International undergraduate and graduate student organization providing educational, mentoring, and peer support for students interested in or now performing basic or clinical psychedelic research.

Website: intercollegiatepsychedelics.net

International Center for Ethnobotanical Education, Research, and Service (ICEERS)

A nonprofit organization dedicated to transforming society's relationship with psychoactive plants.

Website: iceers.org

Microdose

A guide to the business of psychedelics.

Website: microdose.buzz

Multidisciplinary Association for Psychedelic Studies (MAPS)

Nonprofit research, advocacy, and educational organization that develops medical, legal, and cultural contexts for use of psychedelics and marijuana.

Website: maps.org

Psychedelic Grad

A community for up-and-coming psychedelic professionals.

Website: psychedelicgrad.com

The Microdose

A newsletter from the UC Berkeley Center for the Science of Psychedelics.

Website: themicrodose.substack.com

Usona Institute

Conducts and supports pre-clinical and clinical research to further the understanding of the therapeutic effects of psychedelics.

Website: usonainstitute.org

Vaults of Erowid

A member-supported organization providing access to reliable, non-judgmental information about psychoactive plants, chemicals, and related issues. Thousands of trip accounts.

Website: erowid.org.

ACKNOWLEDGMENTS

This book is only possible because of the mentors, teachers, supervisors, colleagues, and friends who have shared their knowledge, wisdom, and kindness with me throughout my life. Among them are Kay Blacker, MD; Frank Cannon; Jim Fadiman, PhD; Daniel X. Friedman, MD; Lucinda Grande, MD; Willis Harman, PhD; John Hopkins, MD; Rakesh Jain, MD; Jiyu Kennett; Haim Kreisel, PhD; Deborah Mash, PhD; Glenn Peake, MD; Eva Petakovic; Clifford Qualls, PhD; Ivan Smith; Rabbi H. Norman Strickman, PhD; Joe Tupin, MD; Norman Wessells, PhD; and Leo Zeff, PhD. The National Institute on Drug Abuse and the Scottish Rite Foundation for Schizophrenia Research provided grant support for my DMT and psilocybin studies. In addition to generous funding, the University of New Mexico General Clinical Research Center also provided an unstintingly supportive research environment. At Ulysses Press, many thanks to my patient and perceptive editors Ashten Evans, Kierra Sondereker, and Scott Calamar. And finally, my heartfelt appreciation to the volunteers in my University of New Mexico studies, as well as the thousands of people who have reached out to share their psychedelic drug experiences with me since then.

ABOUT THE AUTHOR

A native of Los Angeles, Rick Strassman obtained his undergraduate degree in biological sciences from Stanford University and his medical degree from Albert Einstein College of Medicine of Yeshiva University in the Bronx, New York. He trained in general psychiatry at the University of California Davis Medical Center in Sacramento, and took a clinical psychopharmacology research fellowship at the University of California San Diego. At the University of New Mexico School of Medicine, his clinical research team discovered the first known function of melatonin in humans. Between 1990 and 1995, he performed the first new US clinical research with psychedelic drugs in a generation, studying DMT and psilocybin. From 1995 to 2008, Dr. Strassman practiced general psychiatry in community mental health and the private sectors.

Author or coauthor of nearly fifty peer-reviewed papers, Dr. Strassman has served as guest editor and reviewer for numerous scientific journals, and consulted to academic, government, nonprofit, and for-profit entities. His 2001 book *DMT: The Spirit Molecule* has been translated into fourteen languages and is the basis of a successful independent documentary of the same name. Dr. Strassman coauthored *Inner Paths to Outer Space* (2008), and is the author of *DMT and the Soul of Prophecy* (2014), and the novel *Joseph Levy Escapes Death* (2019). He is currently Adjunct Associate Professor of Psychiatry at the University of New Mexico School of Medicine and lives in Gallup, New Mexico.